THE
DENTAL
ASSISTANT'S
GUIDE

Mastering Dental Care Excellence

:Corina-Dean; .McCabe-Jones:

To order additional copies of this book, contact:
Xlibris
844-714-8691
www.Xlibris.com
Orders@Xlibris.com

ISBN: Softcover   979-8-3694-0844-5
             EBook   979-8-3694-0843-8

Library of Congress Control Number: 2023918597

Print information available on the last page

Rev. date: 01/18/2024

Table of Contents

Dear Reader,

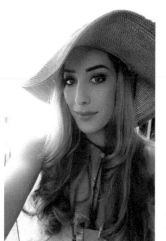

Welcome to my manual, and thank you for choosing to embark on this dental journey with me. My name is Corina Jones, and I am an experienced Registered Dental Assistant with a passion for helping children achieve optimal oral health. Over my 21-year career, I have had the privilege of working in various dental fields, gaining expertise in front office, back office, office management, oral sedation, hospital settings, and both general and pediatric dentistry.

I discovered my true calling in working with children, an area that has always held a special place in my heart. It brings me immense joy to contribute to their oral healthcare needs. Along this path, I have been fortunate to work alongside exceptional dental professionals who have shaped my knowledge, skills, and dedication. I owe a debt of gratitude to my esteemed mentors, Levi Palmer Pediatric Specialist DDS, and Mark Cooper DDS, whose guidance has been invaluable in shaping my understanding of the intricacies of dentistry.

While my local experiences have been fulfilling, I felt a calling to extend my knowledge globally. I have embarked on international endeavors to share my expertise with aspiring dentists and make a difference in the oral healthcare of children worldwide. This Dental Manual is a reflection of my unwavering commitment and passion for the field.

Designed to cater to dental professionals, parents, and caregivers, this comprehensive guide addresses the unique challenges involved in treating both adults and children. By emphasizing the significance of early dental care and preventive measures, we can navigate the complexities of pediatric dentistry and ensure the health and well-being of future generations.

Once again, thank you for choosing this manual as your companion. I am delighted to have you join me on this journey toward excellence in dental care. Together, let's make a difference in the lives of both adults and children and strive for a healthier, happier future.

Warm regards,

:Corina-Dean; .McCabe Jones:

LESSON 1
Direct supervision and indirect supervision

A dental assistant's role is often defined by their direct supervisor and the regulations set by their state's dental board. Here's an explanation of direct supervision and indirect supervision, along with the duties that a dental assistant (DA) and a Registered Dental Assistant (RDA) can perform:

1. Direct Supervision: In the context of dental assisting, direct supervision means that a licensed dentist is present in the office and is physically present during the procedure. Under direct supervision, a DA or RDA can perform a wider range of duties, including:

    –   Assisting the dentist during procedures, such as handing instruments, operating suction, or holding materials.
    –   Taking and developing dental X-rays under the dentist's instruction.
    –   Preparing and sterilizing instruments and equipment.
    –   Providing patient education and post-operative instructions.
    –   Conducting preliminary oral assessments or screenings.

2. Indirect Supervision: Indirect supervision means that a licensed dentist has given authorization but does not need to be physically present while the dental assistant performs certain tasks. The specific duties that can be performed under indirect supervision may vary depending on state regulations. Some common duties that can be performed under indirect supervision include:

    –   Placing and removing rubber dams.
    –   Placing and removing matrix bands.
    –   Placing and removing temporary restorations.
    –   Placing and removing periodontal dressings.

It's important for dental assistants to work within their scope of practice and follow the guidelines provided by their state's dental board. While it's understandable that some doctors may ask you to perform tasks outside of your scope, it's essential to prioritize patient safety and adhere to legal and ethical boundaries.

Performing tasks beyond your authorized scope can have serious consequences, including legal and professional repercussions. If a doctor requests something outside of your scope, it's important to communicate your limitations respectfully and seek clarification or guidance from your direct supervisor or the dental board if necessary.

Remember, patient safety and compliance with regulations should always be the top priority, even if means declining a request from a doctor that falls outside of your scope of practice.

Dental Assistant

General Supervision

1. Extra- oral duties of functions specified by the supervising dentist.
2. Operating of dental radiographic equipment for the purpose of oral radiography if the dental assistant has complied with the requirements for Section 1656 of the Business and Profession Code.

Direct Supervision

1. Taking of impressions for diagnostic and opposing models, bleaching trays, temp crowns and bridges, sports guards, and occlusal guards.
2. Application of non- aerosol and non- caustic topical agents.
3. Removal of post- extraction and periodontal dressings.
4. Placement of elastic orthodontic separators.
5. Removal of orthodontic separators.
6. Assisting in the administration pf Nitrous Oxide (N2O) when used as an analgesia or sedation, but shall not start the administration of the gases and shall not adjust the flow of the gases unless instructed to do so by the dentist who shall be present at the patient's chairside at the implementation of these instruction. This regulation shall not be constued to prevent any person from taking appropriate action in the event of a medical emergency.
7. Holding anterior matrices
8. Removal of sutures
9. Taking of intra- oral measurements for orthodontic procedures
10. Seating of adjusted retainers or headgear, including appropriate instructions.
11. Removal of arch wires
12. Removal of ligature ties
13. Application of topical fluoride, after scaling and polishing by the supervising dentist or a registered dental hygienist
14. Placement and removal of rubber dams
15. Placing, wedging and removing of matrices
16. Cure restorative or orthodontic materials in an operative site

Registered Dental Assistant

The Registered Dental Assistant (RDA), a licensed person, may perform all functions listed for the dental assistant under the appropriate supervision, as well as the following:

General Supervision

1. Mouth- mirror inspection of the oral cavity, to include charting of obvious lesions, existing restorations and missing teeth
2. Placement and removal of temporary sedative dressings

Direct Supervision

1. Obtain endodontic cultures
2. Dry canals, previously opened by the supervising dentist, with absorbent points
3. Test pulp vitality
4. Placing bases and liners on sound dentin
5. Removal of cement excess from supragingival surfaces of teeth with hand instrument of floss
6. Examine orthodontic appliances
7. Sizing of crowns, temporary crowns and bands
8. Temporary size, fit, cementation and removal of temporary crowns and removal of orthodontic bands
9. Intra- oral fabrication of temp crowns
10. Placement of wire orthodontic separators
11. Placement of post- extraction and periodontal dressings
12. Coronal polishing (evidence of satisfactory completion of Board approved course of instruction in this function must be submitted to the Board prior to any performance thereof.)
13. Take bite registration for diagnostic models for case study
14. Supragingival cement removal on teeth under orthodontic treatment with an ultrasonic scaler after completion of an approved course.
15. Apply and activate bleaching agents with non- laser light- curing devices.

Info on can be found at www.dbc.ca.gov

Legal and Ethical Considerations

1. HIPAA (Health Portability and Accountability): HIPAA is a federal law that protects privacy and security of patients' health information. It establishes standards for the electronic exchange, privacy, and security of health information. Dental practices must comply with HIPAA regulations by implementing safeguards to protect patient information and ensuring the confidentiality of sensitive data.

2. Confidentiality and Privacy Rules: Dental practitioners have a legal and ethical obligation to maintain patient confidentiality and privacy. Patient records, including medical history, treatment plans, and financial records should be kept secure and only accessed by authorized individuals. Sharing patient information without proper consent or for non-medical purposes is strictly prohibited.

3. Informed Consent: When providing dental treatment, obtaining informed consent from patients informed consent involves the proposed treatment, its risks and benefits, alternatives, and expected outcomes. Patients should have a clear understanding of their active participation in decision-making.

4. Compliance with Laws: Dental practices must comply with various legal requirements, including state laws and regulations governing dental practice, professional conduct, and advertising. These laws include licensing requirements, infection control protocols, record-keeping obligations, and guidelines for the use of anesthesia and sedation.

5. Patient Rights: Patients have certain rights regarding their These rights may be the right to access their medical records, the right to privacy and confidentiality, the right to refuse treatment, right to receive clear and accurate information about options, and the right to complain or seek a second opinion if necessary.

It is crucial for dental practitioners and staff to stay updated on current legal and ethical guidelines and regularly review their policies and procedures to ensure compliance. Consulting with legal professionals or dental associations can provide further guidance on specific legal and ethical considerations in dental practice.

Lesson 2

Sterilization and Infection Control Measures

- **Importance of Sterilization:**

Sterilization is crucial in the dental field to ensure the safety and well-being of both patients and dental professionals. Proper sterilization practices help prevent the transmission of infectious diseases and maintain a clean and hygienic environment in the dental office. By effectively sterilizing dental instruments and equipment, the risk of cross-contamination and infection is minimized. This not only protects patients but also establishes trust and professionalism in the dental practice.

- **Significance and Management of Sterilized Dental Products:**

Managing sterilized dental products involves proper storage, handling, and maintenance to ensure their integrity and effectiveness. This includes techniques like proper packaging and labeling of sterilized items, following recommended expiration dates, maintaining sterilization logs, and implementing a system for tracking and monitoring sterilized products. Effective management ensures that sterilized items remain safe and ready for use when needed, reducing the risk of contamination and maintaining high standards of infection control.

- **Comprehensive Breakdown of OSHA/ CDC-required Sterilization Chemicals:**

The Occupational Safety and Health Administration (OSHA) and the Centers for Disease Control (CDC) have specific requirements for sterilization in dental offices. These requirements extend to the use of certain chemicals for sterilizing techniques.

CDC and OSHA Recommendations for Dental Offices Regarding COVID-19 Protocols:

To ensure the safety and well-being of dental offices during the COVID-19 pandemic, the Centers for Disease Control and Prevention (CDC) and the Occupational Safety and Health Administration (OSHA) have provided essential recommendations. These guidelines aim to minimize the transmission of the virus and protect both patients and staff. It is important to stay updated with the latest guidelines as they may evolve over time and to comply with local regulations specific to your area.

CDC Recommendations for Dental Offices:

1. **Infection Prevention and Control Measures:** Implement measures such as proper hand hygiene, respiratory etiquette, and thorough environmental cleaning.
2. **Pre-Appointment Screenings:** Conduct screenings for patients and staff to identify potential COVID-19 cases.
3. **Personal Protective Equipment (PPE):** Ensure that dental healthcare personnel have access to and appropriately use PPE.
4. **Engineering Controls:** Implement physical barriers and proper ventilation to minimize the transmission of respiratory droplets.
5. **Social Distancing:** Practice social distancing in waiting areas and throughout the dental office.
6. **Cleaning and Disinfection:** Enhance protocols for regularly cleaning and disinfecting frequently touched surfaces.
7. **Dental Unit Waterlines:** Implement strategies to manage waterlines and reduce the risk of microbial contamination.
8. **Aerosol-Generating Procedures:** Employ measures to minimize aerosol-generating procedures and utilize appropriate mitigating strategies when performing them.
9. **Patient and Staff Education:** Educate patients and staff about COVID-19 prevention measures, and establish clear communication channels for queries or concerns.
10. **Compliance:** Adhere to local, state, and federal regulations and guidelines.

OSHA Recommendations for Dental Offices:

1. **Infectious Disease Preparedness and Response Plan:** Develop a plan that addresses potential COVID-19 exposure risks and outlines responsive actions.
2. **Hazard Assessment:** Conduct an assessment to identify exposure risks and implement control measures accordingly.
3. **Employee Training:** Provide comprehensive training to employees on infection control protocols and recognizing COVID-19 symptoms.
4. **Personal Protective Equipment (PPE):** Ensure the availability and proper use of PPE, including masks, face shields, gloves, and gowns.
5. **Engineering Controls:** Implement engineering measures such as physical barriers and ventilation systems to reduce exposure risks.
6. **Administrative Controls:** Employ administrative measures like work scheduling and patient flow management to minimize the risk of exposure.

7. **Cleaning and Disinfection:** Enhance cleaning and disinfection practices for all areas of the dental office.
8. **Respiratory Hygiene and Cough Etiquette:** Encourage employees and patients to follow proper respiratory hygiene and cough etiquette.
9. **Monitoring and Updates:** Stay informed about changes in guidance from health authorities and update protocols accordingly.
10. **Compliance:** Adhere to all relevant OSHA standards and regulations.

Stay informed and follow these guidelines diligently to safeguard the health and safety of everyone within dental office settings.

Please remember that these recommendations are subject to change, so it's important to remain updated with the latest guidance from the CDC, OSHA, and local health authorities.

Here are some of the chemicals commonly used in dental sterilization:

- Autoclave: An autoclave is a device that uses steam and pressure to sterilize dental instruments. No additional chemicals are typically required in this process.
- Chemical Sterilants/Disinfectants: OSHA requires the use of Environmental Protection Agency (EPA)-registered disinfectants or sterilants in dental offices to ensure effective disinfection Examples include sodium hypochlorite (commonly known as bleach), hydrogen peroxide, and quaternary ammonium compounds
- Hand Sanitizers: OSHA recommends the use of hand sanitizers containing at least 60% alcohol for effective hand hygiene and infection control in dental offices
- Surface Disinfectants: OSHA mandates the use of appropriate surface disinfectants that are effective against bloodborne pathogens and other microorganisms These may include products containing quaternary ammonium compounds, phenolic compounds, or hydrogen peroxide-based formulations

Operatory Breakdown cleaning and disinfection:

- Begin by donning personal protective equipment, including fluid-resistant body protection, protective eyewear, a mask, and heavy-duty chemical-resistant gloves.
- Dispose of all sharps in the designated operatory sharps containers.
- Inspect contaminated instruments and carefully remove debris using gauze.
- Place appropriate instruments back into cassettes and securely close them.
- Load the tray with all cassettes, loose contaminated instruments, and capsules. Any red bag waste should be placed in the tray's side red bag for disposal.

- Remove all disposable barriers and dispose of garbage in the operatory receptacle.
- Transport the tray carefully to the designated "Dirty" area in the sterilization room.
- Review the instrument processing protocol posted in the "Dirty" area of the sterilization room.
- While still wearing heavy-duty gloves, use a suitable cleaning product to clean the gloves.
- Return to the operatory and start cleaning from the cleanest area behind the operatory chair. Clean all items on countertops and countertops using an appropriate cleaning product. Clean all protective eyewear and face shields.
- Use the designated cleaning product to clean tubing and handpiece attachments on the tray counter.
- Clean the side countertops and all items on the side countertop, including x-ray equipment, writing instruments, and drawer handles.
- Wipe down the patient chair, assistant's chair, and dentist's chair.
- Use the designated cleaning product and clean the heavy-duty gloves.
- Using a suitable disinfectant spray, turn the nozzle to "mist" and apply it to surfaces and items throughout the operatory, ensuring that the treated areas remain wet for the required contact time for effective disinfection.
- Use the designated disinfectant product to disinfect the heavy-duty gloves. Remove the gloves and hang them to dry.
- Wash hands thoroughly with soap and water or use an alcohol-based hand sanitizer.
- Organize and store all countertop items back into cabinets for storage.
- Replace barriers on all computer equipment, handpieces, x-ray head, switches, TV remote, light handles, headrests, etc.
- Flush air and water lines for 2 minutes at the start of each day and for 20 seconds between each patient.
- Flush air and water lines for 2 minutes at the start of each day and for 20 seconds between each patient.

Remember to use the specific products and follow the protocols recommended by your dental office and regulatory guidelines.

How to Sterilize Dental Instruments

Ensuring the cleanliness of dental instruments is of utmost importance to prevent disease transmission and cross-contamination. Patients rely on dental offices to use sterile instruments during their treatment. Although dental offices ask about a patient's health history to be aware of potential diseases, patients may not always provide complete and accurate information.

Sterilization Area:

STEP 1: Bringing Instruments Into the Sterilization Area

After a patient leaves the dental office, the instruments used during the procedure must be taken to the sterilization room. In the sterilization room, there are two sides - the "dirty" side and the "clean" side. The dirty side is where instruments are placed when they need to be cleaned and sterilized.

Step 2: Putting on Personal Protective Gear and Pre-cleaning the Instruments Before starting the cleaning process, the person responsible for instrument cleaning should wear personal protective gear, including exam gloves, a mask, eyewear, and big utility gloves to protect themselves and minimize the risk of infection. The instruments cannot be immediately placed in the sterilizer. There are a few steps to be taken before reaching the sterilization phase. First, rinse the instruments under the sink to remove any saliva and debris. Then, retrieve a container with holes called a cassette from a drawer and place the instruments inside it. Close the cassette and transfer it to the ultrasonic water bath, which helps remove additional debris and saliva. The ultrasonic should be operated for 5-10 minutes, taking care not to leave the instruments in for too long to avoid corrosion or rusting. To properly sterilize instruments, follow these steps:

- After running the ultrasonic to clean the instruments, remove them and rinse them thoroughly under the sink. Dry them well using a towel on the counter. Remember not to put wet instruments into sterilizer bags, as it could cause corrosion or rust.

- Ensure that the instruments are completely dry. Then, choose an appropriate sterilizer package based on the instrument size. If you're packaging them as a procedure set, select the largest package that can accommodate all instruments. Carefully place each instrument into the package to avoid tearing it. If a hole appears, discard that package and use a new one. Once all instruments are in the package, seal the top and label it with the date and initials of the person who packaged them.

Step 3: Getting Instruments Ready for the Sterilizer

- **N**ow, the instruments can be placed in the sterilizer. There are various types of sterilizers available, such as Midmark and Stratum. Put the instruments into the chosen sterilizer. Once the sterilizer is full, start the process. Look for buttons with pictorial labels, usually including a "pouches" button, and press it, followed by the start button.

- When the sterilizer completes its cycle, take out the instruments and place them on the clean side and place date on them then there ready to go in storage Before storing, check the package for any holes If a hole is found, the instruments are no longer sterile and should be re-sterilized Once all instruments are checked and put away Ensuring that each step is performed correctly is crucial to prevent the transfer of germs between patients Once the instruments have undergone rinsing and ultrasonic cleaning, they are ready to be placed in the sterilizer Different types of sterilizers, such as Midmark and Stratum, are commonly used in dental offices Load the instruments into the sterilizer and, when it is full, start the cycle The sterilizer typically has four buttons with pictures; press the "pouches" button and then the "start" button

LESSON 3

Maintenance

Beginning of the Day:

1. Check and replenish dental supplies: Optimal patient care requires adequate availability of dental supplies such as gloves, masks, and sterilization pouches. Checking and replenishing supplies at the beginning of the day ensures they are readily available for daily procedures, reducing any inconvenience or disruptions during patient treatments.
2. Clean and disinfect treatment chairs and surfaces: Infection control and patient safety are top priorities in dental practice. Cleaning and disinfecting treatment chairs and surfaces at the beginning of the day helps maintain a clean and safe environment, reducing the risk of cross-contamination.
3. Prepare dental unit water bottle and flush lines: Dental procedures often require a continuous supply of clean water. Preparing the dental unit water bottle and flushing lines ensures a proper water supply, maintaining the quality and safety of water used during treatments.

Beginning of the Day:

- Fill ultrasonic solution
- Turn on MidMark #1 and #2 and Statim
- Fill water at chairs (water and MicroClean)
- Run water lines for 2 min. Before pt arrives
- Run handpieces for 20 sec. After pt TX and before PT TX begins
- Run Suction lines with cleaner before pts arrives
- Turn on computers / log-in
- Turn on water and Vacuum
- Turn on N2O/ Oxygen tanks
- Check schedule
- Get Trays ready
- Set chairs up for pts
- Date sterilization bags and write #1 or #2 on pouches
    - Check date on cold sterile
    - Clean /Stock
    - Power/ units/ vacuum off

End of the Day:

1. Clean and disinfect handpieces: Handpieces are heavily used during dental procedures and can become contaminated. Proper cleaning and disinfection at the end of the day prevent cross-contamination, ensuring a safe and hygienic working environment.

2. Empty and clean amalgam separator: Amalgam separators collect amalgam waste, preventing it from entering the wastewater system. Regular emptying and cleaning of amalgam separators prevent waste buildup, maintain suction system efficacy, and contribute to environmental protection.

3. Turn off and unplug equipment: Turning off and unplugging equipment at the end of the day reduces energy consumption, lowers the risk of electrical hazards, and promotes equipment longevity.

   – Log off/ Shut Down Computers
   – Thoroughly Clean Lab
   – Clean/ Stock Units Drawers
   – Vacuum/ Sweep clinic
   – Take out Garbage's and Recycle
   – Electronics off
   – Place Curing Lights on chargers
   – Clean/ organize Island in clinic
– **Stock Trays w/ Set- up**

Weekly Maintenance:

1. Check and clean handpieces: Handpieces are crucial tools for dental procedures. Regular cleaning ensures their proper functionality and prevents cross-contamination, maintaining a safe and hygienic environment for both patients and staff.

2. Inspect and clean suction system filters: Suction systems play a vital role in maintaining a clean and saliva-free working area. Regularly inspecting and cleaning the filters prevent clogs, ensuring proper suction and preventing any negative impact on dental procedures.

3. Check and clean autoclave: The autoclave is used for sterilizing dental instruments. Regular maintenance and cleaning are essential to ensure the autoclave's effectiveness in killing bacteria and maintaining high sterilization standards. This helps prevent the spread of infections and prolongs the equipment's lifespan.

4. Inspect waterlines and flush with appropriate cleaning solution: Dental waterlines can accumulate biofilm over time, which can harbor bacteria and compromise water quality. Regular inspections and flushing with appropriate cleaning solutions help prevent biofilm buildup, maintain water quality, and ensure safe water supply for dental procedures.

5. Test emergency equipment (e.g., fire extinguisher, emergency oxygen tank): Emergency equipment is crucial for ensuring the safety of patients and staff. Regular testing of emergency equipment, such as fire extinguishers and emergency oxygen tanks, ensures their readiness in case of emergencies and helps prevent potential hazards

Weekly:

Schedule maintenance of dental chairs, lights, and other equipment as per manufacturer recommendations: Regular maintenance as per manufacturer recommendations helps prevent breakdowns and malfunctions. It ensures optimal performance, extends the lifespan of equipment, and reduces the risk of unexpected failures.

Weekly/Monthly Duties:

- Restock Cavicide wipes and spray bottles
- Check hand sanitizer/soaps
- Refill water bottles
- Drain Gleco Traps (change if full)
- Lube 4-way Suctions
- Thoroughly clean Micro Etcher
- Label and restock retainer cases
- Fold and put away T-shirts
- Lube/ oil/ sterile handpieces
- Drain and maintain MidMark #1 #2 and Statim (Monthly)
- Run and mail out spore test
- Scrub down unit chairs with mild soap
- Thoroughly stock/ clean units
- Check to clean/ change unit traps (Monthly)

Monthly:

1. Calibrate dental x-ray machines: Dental x-ray machines need to be calibrated regularly to ensure accurate radiation exposure and high - quality imaging. Proper

calibration helps prevent underexposure or overexposure to radiation and ensures accurate diagnoses and treatment planning.

2. Inspect and clean compressor unit: Compressors supply air to various dental equipment. Regular inspection and cleaning help maintain proper air pressure, preventing breakdowns and ensuring uninterrupted functionality of dental instruments.

3. **Lubricate handpiece turbines: Handpiece turbines require regular lubrication to prevent overheating and damage. Proper lubrication enhances their lifespan and ensures smooth and efficient operation during dental procedures.**

Inspect and clean ultrasonic cleaner: Ultrasonic cleaners are essential for dental instrument cleaning. Regular inspection and cleaning maintain their cleaning efficacy and prolong their lifespan, allowing for efficient and effective instrument cleaning.

Monthly Check:

– Eyewash Station
– Fire EXT.
– Emergency Kit
– Oxygen
– N2O Tanks

Yearly:

1. Schedule professional maintenance and inspection of equipment: Professional maintenance and inspection provide a comprehensive evaluation of dental equipment and identify potential issues. This helps ensure compliance with regulatory standards, maximize equipment efficiency, and address any potential problems before they become significant.

Documentation is crucial to keep track of maintenance tasks performed. Each task should be documented with initials and a date to indicate completion. This documentation helps maintain an organized record of upkeep, enables tracking equipment performance, and aids in addressing any potential issues efficiently.

LESSON 4

Anatomy of Teeth: Primary and Permanent:

– Tooth Structure: Understanding the anatomy of primary (deciduous) and permanent teeth is crucial for dental assistants. Here is a detailed explanation of tooth structure, including tooth numbering systems and identification based on location and characteristics:

Tooth Structure:

1. **Crown:** The crown is the visible part of the tooth above the gumline. It is covered by enamel, which is the hardest and most mineralized tissue in the human body.
2. Root: The root is the part of the tooth that is embedded in the jawbone. It anchors the tooth in place.
3. **Enamel**: Enamel is the outermost layer of the tooth's crown. It is highly mineralized and protects the inner layers of the tooth.
4. **Dentin:** Dentin lies beneath the enamel and forms the majority of the tooth structure. It is calcified tissue that is less hard than enamel but still provides support and strength to the tooth.
5. **Pulp:** The dental pulp is located in the center of the tooth. It contains nerves, blood vessels, and connective tissue. The pulp provides nourishment to the tooth and plays a role in sensory perception.
6. **Cementum:** Cementum covers the root surface of the tooth and helps to anchor the tooth to the jawbone. It is not as hard as enamel.
7. **Periodontal ligament (PDL):** The PDL is a group of fibers that attach the tooth root to the jawbone, providing stability and acting as a shock absorber.
8. Alveolar bone: The alveolar bone is the specialized bone that surrounds and supports the teeth. It holds the teeth in their sockets.

Tooth Numbering Systems:

There are two common tooth numbering systems used in dentistry: the Universal Numbering System and the Palmer Notation Method.

1. **Universal Numbering System**: This system assigns a number to each tooth, starting from the upper right third molar as "1" and continuing in a clockwise direction until reaching the upper left third molar as "16". The numbering continues to the lower left

third molar as "17", and then proceeds in a clockwise direction until ending at the lower right third molar as "32".

2. **Palmer Notation Method:** This method uses symbols to represent the quadrant of the mouth and a number for the tooth. The mouth is divided into four quadrants: the upper right (UR), upper left (UL), lower left (LL), and lower right (LR). Each tooth is assigned a number from 1 to 8, with 1 being the central incisor and 8 being the third molar. For example, the upper right second molar would be represented as UR7.

Tooth Identification:

Tooth identification involves recognizing specific teeth based on their location and characteristics. Here are some key identifiers for each tooth:

1. **Incisors:** Incisors are the front teeth (central incisors and lateral incisors) in both the primary and permanent dentitions. They are typically smaller and have a sharp, thin edge for cutting food.
2. **Canines (Cuspids):** Canines are located on either side of the incisors. They have a single cusp and a pointed shape, making them useful for tearing and grasping food. Premolars (Bicuspids): Premolars are found behind the canines. They have two cusps and play a role in crushing and grinding food.
3. Molars: Molars are the flattest and largest teeth in the mouth. They are used for chewing and grinding food. The primary dentition typically has four molars, while the permanent dentition has eight molars (including the wisdom teeth).

Tooth identification can also be based on a tooth's position within a quadrant and its relation to neighboring teeth. The terms used include mesial (toward the midline), distal (away from the midline), buccal/ labial (toward the cheek or lips), lingual (toward the tongue), and occlusal (the chewing surface of the posterior teeth). It's important for dental assistants to understand tooth structure, numbering systems, and tooth identification to effectively communicate with the dentist and accurately record findings during dental examinations and treatments.

3. Supernumerary teeth, also known as hyperdontia, are extra teeth that can develop in the oral cavity. They can occur in addition to the normal set of 32 permanent teeth or even in the primary dentition (baby teeth).

Supernumerary teeth can take various forms, such as small, malformed, or fully developed, resembling regular teeth. They can appear anywhere in the dental arch, but they commonly occur in the front region of the upper jaw (maxilla).

When it comes to numbering supernumerary teeth, the internationally recognized numbering system used in dentistry is called the Universal Numbering System. In this system, each tooth is assigned a unique number for identification. The numbering starts from the right maxillary third molar (tooth number 1), then moves around the upper arch to the left third molar (tooth number 16), and continues with the lower arch from the left third molar (tooth number 17) to the right third molar (tooth number 32).

For supernumerary teeth, they are usually assigned numbers beyond the existing dental arch. For example, if a supernumerary tooth is found between the upper right central incisor (tooth number 8) and the upper right lateral incisor (tooth number 9), it may be labeled as tooth number 8A. If another extra tooth is found between the upper left central incisor (tooth number 9) and the upper left lateral incisor (tooth number 10), it may be labeled as tooth number 9A.

It's important to note that the numbering of supernumerary teeth may vary depending on the dental professional and the specific case. Dentists and oral surgeons may use alternative numbering systems or simply describe the location of the supernumerary teeth without assigning a specific number.

4. If you suspect that you have supernumerary teeth or any concerns about your dental health, it's always best to consult a dentist or oral health professional for a proper examination and diagnosis.

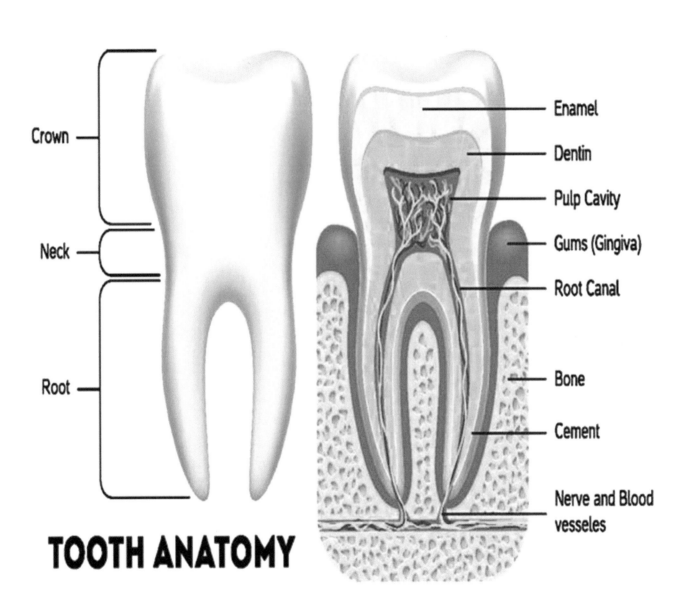

Crown

Neck

Root

Enamel

Dentin

Pulp Cavity

Gums (Gingiva)

Root Canal

Bone

Cement

Nerve and Blood vesseles

TOOTH ANATOMY

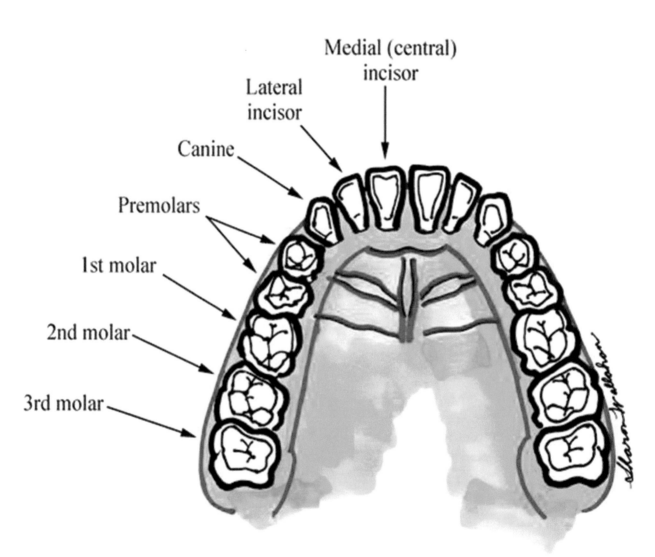

Medial (central)
incisor

Lateral
incisor

Canine

Premolars

1st molar

2nd molar

3rd molar

The stages of tooth decay

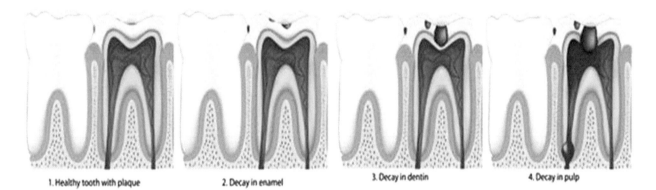

1. Healthy tooth with plaque   2. Decay in enamel   3. Decay in dentin   4. Decay in pulp

Primary (Baby Teeth)

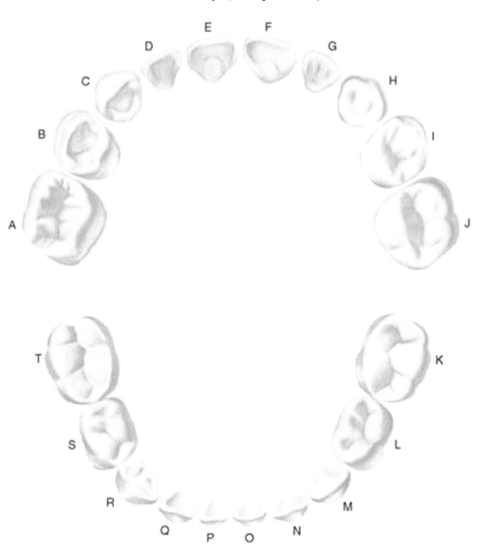

Universal

THE INTERNATIONAL TOOTH NUMBERING SYSTEM

UPPER RIGHT

1. 3rd Molar (wisdom tooth)
2. 2nd Molar (12-year molar)
3. 1st Molar (6-year molar)
4. 2nd Bicuspid (2nd premolar)
5. 1st Bicuspid (1st premolar)
6. Cuspid (canine/eye tooth)
7. Lateral incisor
8. Central incisor

UPPER LEFT

9. Central incisor
10. Lateral incisor
11. Cuspid (canine/eye tooth)
12. 1st Bicuspid (1st premolar)
13. 2nd Bicuspid (2nd premolar)
14. 1st Molar (6-year molar)
15. 2nd Molar (12-year molar)
16. 3rd Molar (wisdom tooth)

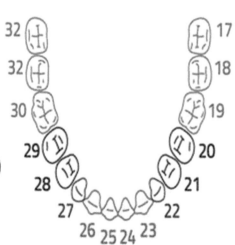

LOWER RIGHT

25. Central incisor
26. Lateral incisor
27. Cuspid (canine/eye tooth)
28. 1st Bicuspid (1st premolar)
29. 2nd Bicuspid (2nd premolar)
30. 1st Molar (6-year molar)
31. 2nd Molar (12-year molar)
32. 3rd Molar (wisdom tooth)

LOWER LEFT

25. 3rd Molar (wisdom tooth)
26. 2nd Molar (12-year molar)
27. 1st Molar (6-year molar)
28. 2nd Bicuspid (2nd premolar)
29. 1st Bicuspid (1st premolar)
30. Cuspid (canine/eye tooth)
31. Lateral incisor
32. Central incisor

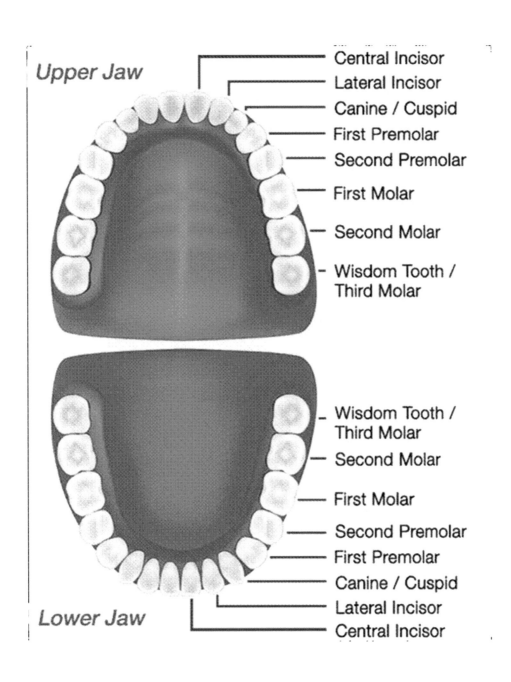

Upper Jaw

Central Incisor
Lateral Incisor
Canine / Cuspid
First Premolar
Second Premolar
First Molar
Second Molar
Wisdom Tooth / Third Molar

Wisdom Tooth / Third Molar
Second Molar
First Molar
Second Premolar
First Premolar
Canine / Cuspid
Lateral Incisor
Central Incisor

Lower Jaw

Buccal

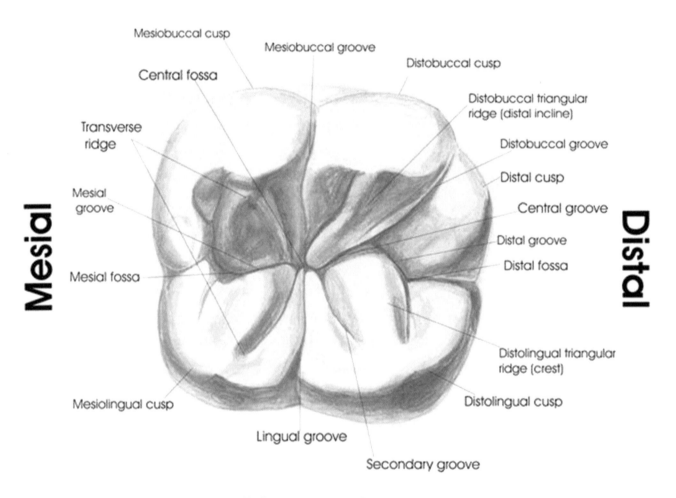

Mesiobuccal cusp

Mesiobuccal groove

Distobuccal cusp

Central fossa

Distobuccal triangular
ridge (distal incline)

Transverse
ridge

Distobuccal groove

Distal cusp

Mesial
groove

Central groove

Distal groove

Mesial fossa

Distal fossa

Mesial

Distal

Distolingual triangular
ridge (crest)

Mesiolingual cusp

Distolingual cusp

Lingual groove

Secondary groove

Lingual

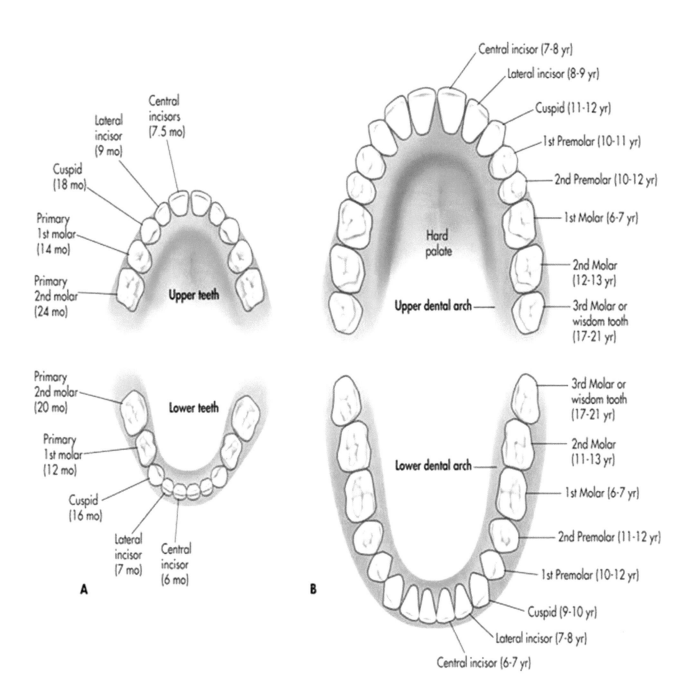

Central incisors (7.5 mo)

Lateral incisor (9 mo)

Cuspid (18 mo)

Primary 1st molar (14 mo)

Primary 2nd molar (24 mo)

Upper teeth

Primary 2nd molar (20 mo)

Lower teeth

Primary 1st molar (12 mo)

Cuspid (16 mo)

Lateral incisor (7 mo)

Central incisor (6 mo)

A

Central incisor (7-8 yr)

Lateral incisor (8-9 yr)

Cuspid (11-12 yr)

1st Premolar (10-11 yr)

2nd Premolar (10-12 yr)

1st Molar (6-7 yr)

2nd Molar (12-13 yr)

3rd Molar or wisdom tooth (17-21 yr)

Hard palate

Upper dental arch

3rd Molar or wisdom tooth (17-21 yr)

2nd Molar (11-13 yr)

1st Molar (6-7 yr)

2nd Premolar (11-12 yr)

1st Premolar (10-12 yr)

Lower dental arch

Cuspid (9-10 yr)

Lateral incisor (7-8 yr)

Central incisor (6-7 yr)

B

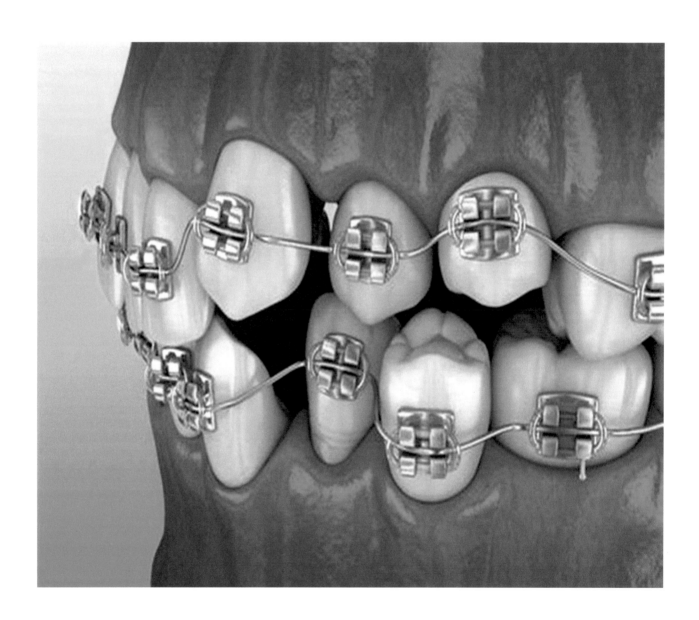

LESSON 5

Empowering Patients: Education and Dental Care

As a dental assistant, it is essential to effectively educate patients and their parents about dental hygiene at home, how to handle dental emergencies, maintain proper nutrition, and understand the importance of home oral care. This section will provide guidance on teaching the new dental assistant how to educate patients and parents on these important topics.

1. Dental Hygiene at Home:

1.1 Importance:

Dental hygiene at home plays a crucial role in maintaining oral health and preventing dental issues such as cavities and gum disease. Educating patients and parents about proper home care empowers them to take responsibility for their oral health.

1.2 Teaching Points:

- Demonstrate and explain proper toothbrushing techniques, emphasizing the importance of brushing for at least two minutes, twice a day.
- Educate patients and parents about the correct method of flossing to remove plaque and food particles from between teeth.(I always tell them floss the ones you want to keep.)
- Explain the benefits of using mouthwash as a supplementary step for maintaining fresh breath and reducing the risk of oral infections.
- Discuss the importance of replacing toothbrushes every three to four months or sooner if the bristles become frayed.

Brushing

Holding brush at 45 angle, brush in short back and forth motions on the outer surfaces of the teeth. Don't scrub.

Use back and forth motion for chewing surfaces.

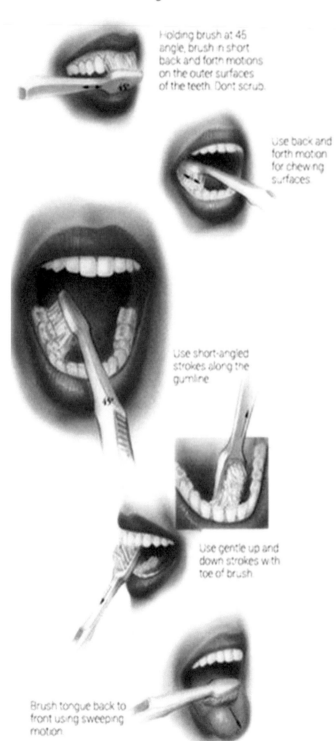

Use short-angled strokes along the gumline.

Use gentle up and down strokes with toe of brush.

Brush tongue back to front using sweeping motion.

Flossing

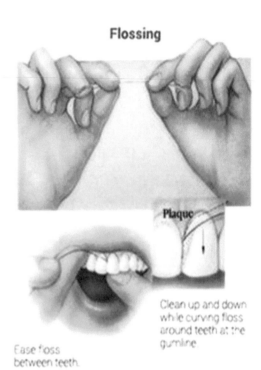

Plaque

Ease floss between teeth.

Clean up and down while curving floss around teeth at the gumline.

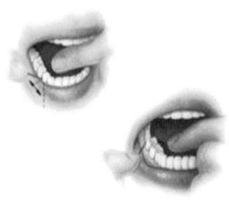

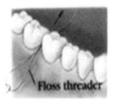

Floss under a bridge using a floss threader.

Floss threader

Floss

2. Dental Emergencies:

2.1 Importance:

Dental emergencies can occur unexpectedly, and knowing how to handle them properly can minimize pain, prevent complications, and provide timely care.

2.2 Teaching Points

Instruct the dental assistant to explain to patients and parents the different types of dental emergencies, such as toothaches, dental trauma, and knocked- out teeth.

- Provide information on immediate actions to take in case of dental emergencies, such as applying cold compresses for swelling, using over-the- counter pain relievers, and preserving knocked-out teeth in milk or saliva until professional help is available.
- Stress the significance of contacting the dentist promptly for guidance and to schedule an emergency appointment.
- Emphasize the importance of a balanced diet rich in fruits and vegetables, whole grains, lean proteins, and dairy products for the overall health of teeth and gums
- Explain the negative impact of excessive consumption of sugary and acidic foods and beverages on oral health, leading to tooth decay and erosion.
- Educate patients and parents on the benefits of drinking water and avoiding sugary drinks.
- Provide resources, such as educational brochures or website recommendations, to further support and reinforce the importance of proper nutrition..

3. Home Oral Care:

3.1 Importance:

- Consistent home oral care routines are vital for maintaining oral health between dental visits and preventing dental problems.

3.2 Teaching Points:

- Demonstrate proper brushing and flossing techniques, emphasizing the importance of cleaning all tooth surfaces and reaching inter dental spaces.
- Encourage patients and parents to establish a regular dental care routine, including brushing at least twice a day and flossing daily.

- Recommend the use of fluoride toothpaste to strengthen teeth and reduce the risk of cavities.
- Discuss the importance of regular dental check-ups and cleanings to monitor oral health and address any issues promptly.

the importance of home oral care, dental assistants empower patients to make informed decisions and take responsibility for their oral health. Continuous education and support contribute to long-term oral well-being and overall health

Dental Terminology Kid-friendly Terminology

Nitrous Oxide or Oxygen - Magic Air or Laughing Gas

Nitrous Mask (N202 mask) - Miss Piggy's Nose, Power Ranger, or Astronaut Nose

Water Rinse - Tooth Shower

Air or Suction - Wind, Vacuum, or Straw

Injection or Shot - Balloon Medicine

Cavities - Cavity Bugs or Sugar Bugs

X-ray - Picture

X-ray Unit - Camera

Leaded Apron - Apron, Cape, or Blanket

Mouth Mirror - Tooth Mirror

Explorer - Tooth Counter

Extraction - Wiggle Out

Rubber Dam - Tooth Umbrella or Raincoat

Rubber Dam Clamp - Tooth Ring

Topical Anesthetic - Special Lotion, Sleepy Gel, or Tickle

Gel Bite block - Pillow

Composites or Fillings - Paint, Mouth Star or Tooth Star

Prophy Angle - Tooth Tickler or Special Toothbrush

Scaler - Tooth Scraper

Fluoride Foam - Tooth Bubble Bath or Tooth Vitamins

Curing Light - Magic Wand or Flashlight

LESSON 6

Common Pediatric Oral Habits and Breaking Them

Chapter 6 explores the most common pediatric oral habits, their impact on oral health, and effective strategies to break these habits. We'll discuss how dentists can assist in the process and the education behind habit cessation. Understanding these habits and their consequences will highlight the significance of early intervention for optimal oral health in children.

1. Thumb Sucking:

1.1 Habit and Consequences:

Thumb sucking is a common instinctive habit that provides comfort and security to young children. However, prolonged thumb sucking can lead to dental issues such as misalignment of teeth, open bite, and speech problems.

1.2 Breaking the Habit:

Breaking the thumb-sucking habit requires patience and encouragement. Parents can:

Provide positive reinforcement and praise when the child refrains from thumb sucking.

Identify triggers and find alternative activities or toys to divert their attention.

Engage the child in discussions about the importance of stopping the habit for a healthy smile.

Consult with the dentist, who can provide additional guidance and interventions, such as applying a habit-breaking dental appliance.

2. Pacifier Use:

2.1 Habit and Consequences:

Similar to thumb sucking, pacifier use provides children with comfort. However, excessive use can lead to dental issues such as misalignment, dental arch deformities, and speech problems.

2.2 Breaking the Habit:

Breaking the pacifier habit requires a gradual approach. Parents can:

- **Encourage the child to use the pacifier less frequently during the day.**
- **Substitute the pacifier with other comforting objects like a stuffed animal or blanket.**
- **Limit pacifier use to specific times, such as bedtime.**
- **Praise the child when they voluntarily give up the pacifier.**
- **Consult with the dentist, who can provide guidance and support throughout the process.**

3. Tongue Thrusting:

3.1 Habit and Consequences:

Tongue thrusting is the habit of pushing the tongue against or between the teeth during swallowing or speaking. This can lead to improper alignment of teeth, open bite, and speech difficulties.

3.2 Breaking the Habit:

Breaking the tongue thrusting habit may require professional intervention and dental guidance. Techniques to consider include:

- **Implementing proper swallowing techniques through exercises and speech therapy.**
- **Using oral appliances or orthodontic treatment to correct tongue posture.**
- **Working closely with the dentist to monitor progress and create a customized treatment plan.**

4. Lip Biting or Lip Sucking:

4.1 Habit and Consequences:

Lip biting or lip sucking can lead to misalignment of teeth and potential trauma to the lips.

4.2 Breaking the Habit:

To break the habit of lip biting or sucking, parents and dentists can:

- Identify triggers and substitute the habit with another form of self-soothing, such as chewing sugarless gum or using a straw.
- Educate the child about the potential consequences of lip biting and involve them in the decision to break the habit.
- Utilize behavioral techniques and positive reinforcement to encourage the child to stop the habit.
- Seek professional guidance from the dentist to address any underlying causes or recommend appropriate treatment.

Understanding common pediatric oral habits and their consequences is integral to maintaining optimal oral health in children. Breaking these habits requires a collaborative effort between parents, children, and dental professionals. Dentists play a vital role in providing education, support, and customized interventions to help children break harmful habits. Early intervention and consistent guidance contribute to the long-term oral well-being and overall development of children.

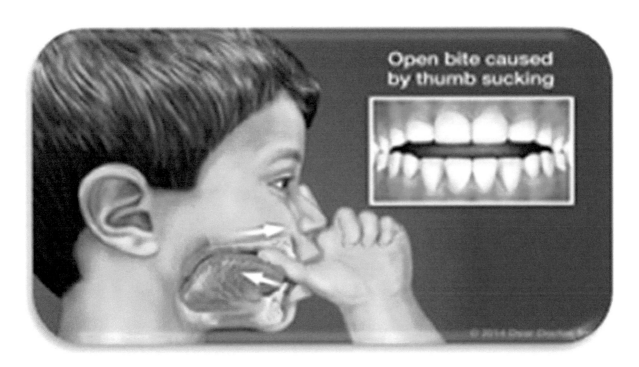

Open bite caused by thumb sucking

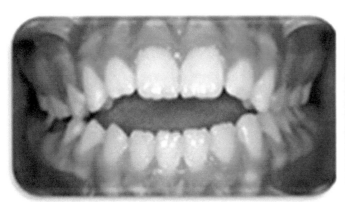

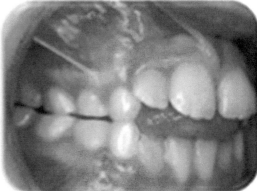

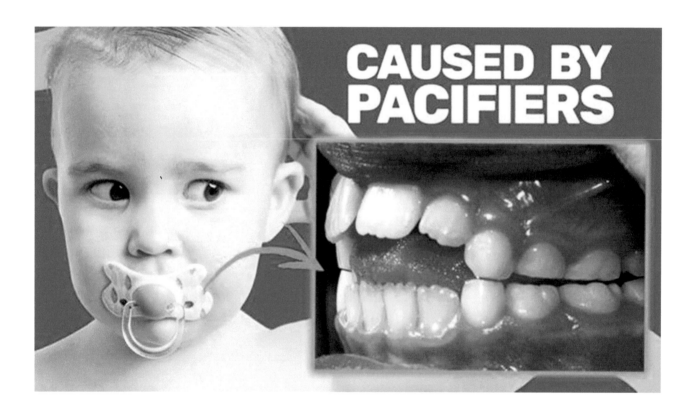

CAUSED BY PACIFIERS

Tongue Thrusting

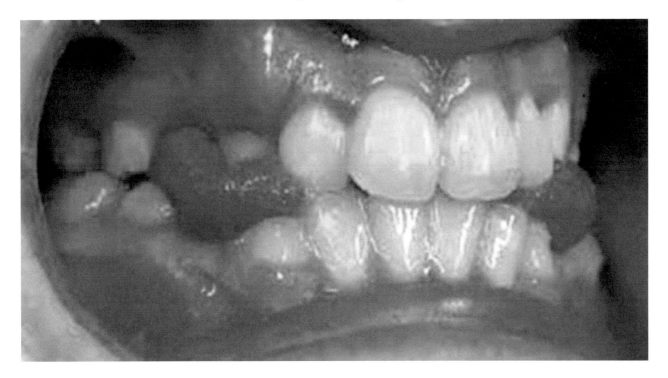

Lip Biting

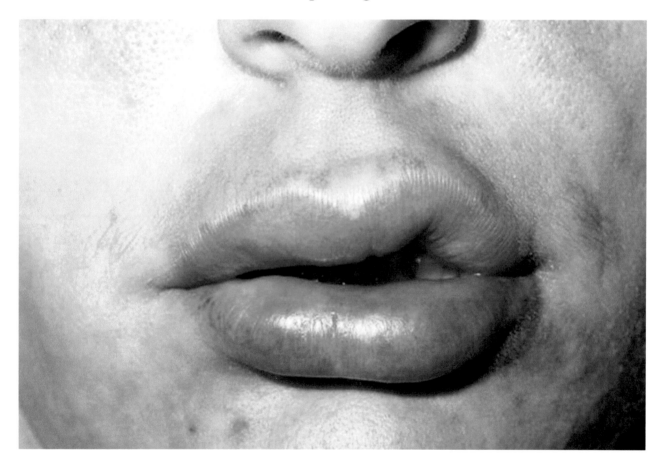

LESSON 7

Special Pediatric Dental Procedures

In this chapter, we will explore the world of special pediatric dental procedures, focusing on essential treatments such as sealants, space maintainers, pediatric partials, and retainers. We will dive into their importance, why they may be needed, and the tools Dentists use to perform these procedures effectively. Understanding these procedures will empower parents and caregivers to make informed decisions and ensure optimal oral health for their children.

1. **Dental Sealants:**

1.1 Importance:

Dental sealants play a crucial role in preventing tooth decay, especially in children who are more prone to developing cavities. As a thin protective coating applied to the chewing surfaces of the back teeth, sealants act as a barrier, blocking food particles and harmful bacteria from settling into the grooves and pits of the teeth. By sealing off these vulnerable areas, sealants significantly reduce the risk of cavities.

1.2 Procedure:

The dental sealant procedure is painless, non-invasive, and completed in a single dental visit. The dentist will thoroughly clean and dry the teeth before applying the sealant material. This liquid resin is carefully painted onto the teeth and bonds to the enamel, creating a shield against decay. A special curing light is then used to harden the sealant, ensuring its durability.

Sealants

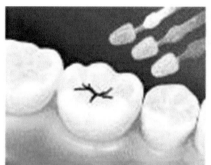

1. Shade selection

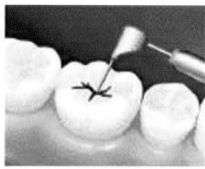

2. Preparation

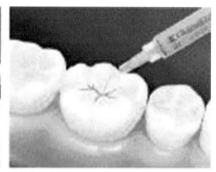

3. Etching

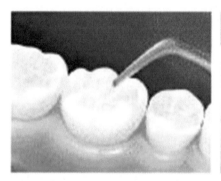

4. Cleaning and dry

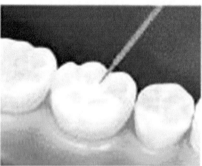

5. Bonding

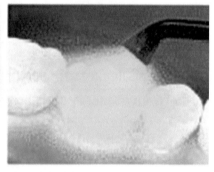

6. Light Curing (20sec)

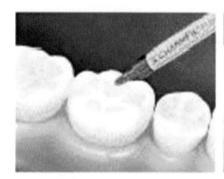

7. Filling

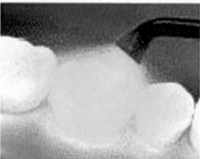

8. Light Curing

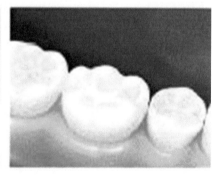

9. Polishing

2. Space Maintainers:

2.1 Importance:

When a primary (baby) tooth is lost prematurely due to decay or trauma, nearby teeth may shift into the empty space, leading to future orthodontic problems. Space maintainers are dental appliances designed to hold the surrounding teeth in place, preventing their movement and guiding the eruption of permanent teeth in their correct positions. By preserving space, these devices help avoid the need for more extensive orthodontic treatment later on.

2.2 Procedure:

Space maintainers are custom-made by the dentist to fit a child's unique dental arch. The device is typically composed of metal wires or acrylic material and can be removable or fixed, depending on the specific case. The dentist will carefully place and adjust the space maintainer, ensuring comfort and effectiveness in maintaining the space until the permanent tooth erupts naturally.

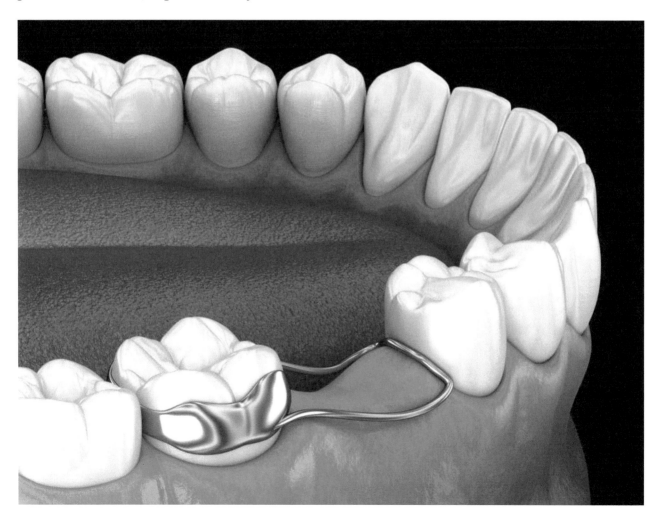

3. **Pediatric Partials:**

3.1 Importance:

Pediatric partial dentures are removable dental appliances designed to replace multiple missing teeth in children. These prosthetic devices are crucial for restoring proper speech, chewing function, and preserving the natural alignment of adjacent teeth. Pediatric partials not only enhance a child's overall oral health but also contribute to their self-esteem and confidence.

3.2 Procedure:

The process for obtaining pediatric partials involves several steps. The dentist will first take impressions of the child's mouth to create an accurate model. The pediatric partial denture is carefully designed and constructed to match the natural appearance of the child's teeth. The dentist will then ensure proper fit and make any necessary adjustments to ensure comfort and functionality.

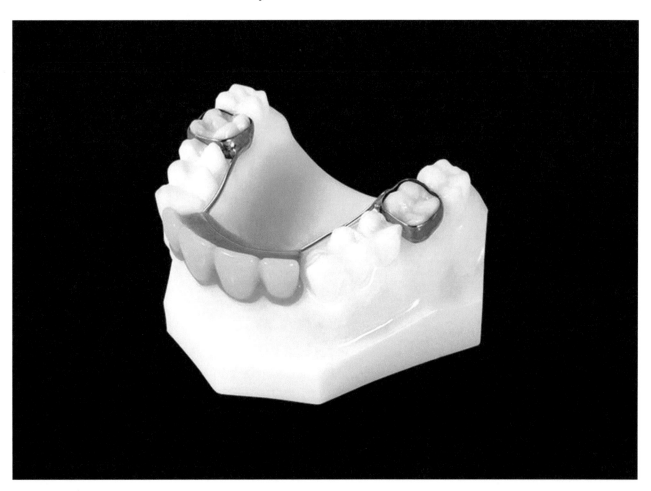

4. **Retainers:**

4.1 Importance:

After orthodontic treatment, retainers play a vital role in maintaining the corrected alignment of teeth. Retainers help prevent teeth from shifting back into their previous positions and offer long-term stability to the orthodontic results obtained. Compliance with retainer wear is crucial to ensuring the success of orthodontic treatment.

4.2 Procedure:

Retainers can be removable or fixed, depending on the specific situation. Removable retainers are often made of clear plastic or wire, and they need to be worn as prescribed by the orthodontist. Fixed retainers, on the other hand, are bonded to the back of the teeth and provide a convenient and constant retention solution.

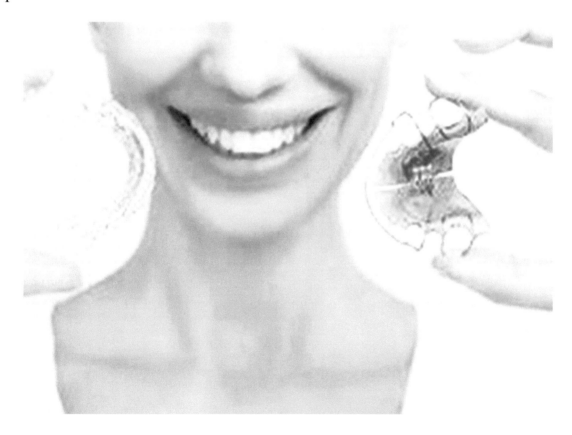

Special pediatric dental procedures such as sealants, space maintainers, pediatric partials, and retainers are crucial for optimizing a child's oral health and development. Understanding their importance and the procedures involved empowers parents and caregivers to make informed decisions in coordination with their dentist or orthodontist. By proactively addressing these dental needs, we ensure the long-term oral well-being of our children.

LESSON 8

Hand-Over-Hand Instrument Technique

Four handed dentistry or hand over hand instrument techniques in the dental field are a fundamental part of dental assisting. It involves using a specific grip and motion to handle dental instruments effectively.

"Hand over hand instrument techniques in dentistry refer to a method of holding and manipulating dental instruments. It involves grasping the instrument with one hand while stabilizing it with the other hand. This grip allows for precise control and reduces the risk of slippage or injury. By using a fluid motion, you'll be able to assist the dentist in performing various procedures accurately and efficiently. Practice and experience will help you develop the necessary dexterity and coordination for this technique." Four-handed dentistry, also known as the hand over hand technique, has been a standard practice in the dental field for several decades. It was developed in the early 20th century as a way to improve efficiency and productivity during dental procedures.

The concept of four-handed dentistry originated from the industrial efficiency principles introduced by Frederick Winslow Taylor in the late 19th century. In the early 1900s, dental professionals began applying these principles to dental practice to streamline procedures and enhance patient care.

The term "four-handed dentistry" refers to the coordinated teamwork between the dentist and dental assistant during procedures. The dentist focuses on performing the treatment, while the dental assistant assists by passing instruments, maintaining a clear field of view, and providing support to the patient.

1. Maintain proper positioning: Stand or sit close to the dentist's working area, ensuring good visibility of the field and maintaining a comfortable working posture.

2. Anticipate the dentist's needs: Pay close attention to the procedure being performed and anticipate the next instrument required. This will help streamline the process and make it smoother for the dentist.

3. Select the instrument: Identify the instrument needed based on the procedure and choose the correct size or type. Ensure that it is clean and free of any debris.

4. Orient the instrument correctly: Hold the instrument properly in your dominant hand with a firm yet comfortable grip. The working end of the instrument, such as the pliers or handle, should be facing in the same direction as the dentist's hand when they receive it.

5. Hand over the instrument: Use the hand-over-hand technique to ensure a smooth transfer of the instrument. Start by placing the instrument in the palm of the dentist's hand, ensuring proper alignment. Then, gently release your grip as the dentist gains control of the instrument.

6. Tips for effective communication: Use simple verbal cues or gestures to alert the dentist about the instrument being handed over. For example, you can say, "Explorer, ready?" or use a non -verbal cue, such as nodding your head or pointing to the instrument.

7. Be proactive: As you become more familiar with the procedures and the dentist's preferences, try to anticipate their needs even before they ask for the instrument. This will make the workflow more efficient and help establish a stronger working dynamic.

Remember, open communication and familiarity with the dentist's preferred techniques are key elements in successfully implementing the hand over hand instrument technique. Over time, as you gain experience, you will become more proficient in providing instruments efficiently and intuitively.

Your goal is to know what your Dr. wants before they do. A dental assistant's role is to keep the flow going,if the Dr has to stop so you can go get something that puts everyone behind.. The Dr should never have to take his eyes off the tooth he is working on because a good assent already has the next instrument ready to place in his hand before he even thinks about it. I always tell my kids "When you fail to prepare you prepare to fail."Think of that every time you are setting up your operator room and I promise after some practice you will always be prepared.

LESSON 9

Instrument Identification and tray set up

- Familiarize yourself with the various dental instruments commonly used in dental procedures.

The basic instruments used in dental procedures for beginners include and tray set up:

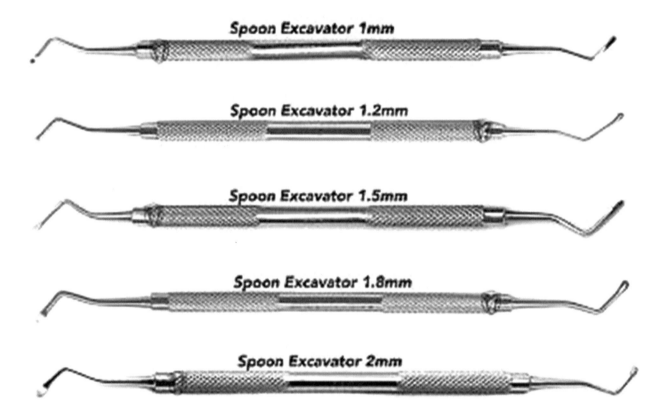

Basic Tray Set- Up and instruments

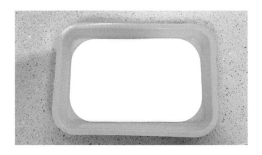

Instrument: Dental Tray

Function: To provide an area specific for instruments

Characteristics: Different designs for different procedures, hygiene tray, operative tray, surgical tray.

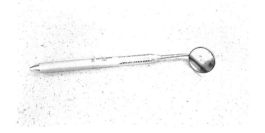

Instrument: Mouth Mirror

Function: To provide indirect vision to retract lips, cheeks, and tongue to reflect light into the mouth.

Characteristics: Accurate image from flat surface mirrors, image magnified with concave mirrors.

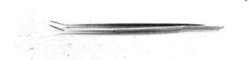

Instrument: Cotton Forceps

Function: To grasp and/ or transfer material in and out of the oral cavity.

Characteristics: Plain or serrated tips variety of sizes, angled tip.

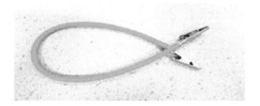

Instrument: Bib holder

Function: To attach the patient bib around the patient's neck.

Characteristics: Disposable snap / adhesive clips Alligator clip (not disposable)

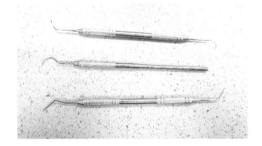

Instrument: Explorers

Function: To examine teeth for decay (caries), calculus, furcation, or canals and other anomalies

Characteristics: Pointed tips: sharp, thin and flexible

- **Pigtail   2. Shepherds   3. Orbin**

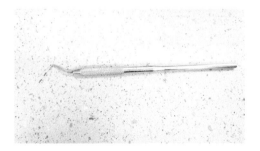

Instrument: Perioprobe

Function: An instrument with incremental marks on the tip to measure the periodontal pockets

Characteristics: Designed with different increments, 1 mm, 3mm, PSR probe

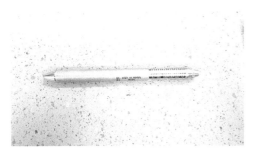

Instrument: Instrument Handles

Function: Handles for detachable instrument, heads screw into handle

Characteristics: mouth mirror

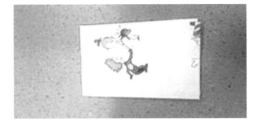

Instrument: Patient Bib

Function: To prevent materials, debris, fluids from contacting the patient

Characteristics: Differs in colors, shapes and designs; has a protective liquid barrier side and absorbent side

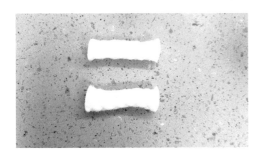

Instrument: Cotton Rolls

Function: To isolate teeth and absorb saliva act as a protective tissue barrier, aid in endodontic diagnostics

Characteristics: Fluid absorbent roll- 1 in long

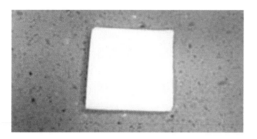

Instrument: 2X2 gauze

Function: absorbent cloth, aid in homeostasis, clean instruments, used in all aspects of dentistry

Characteristics: 2x2 inches in size, white, thinly/ thick woven absorbent fiber

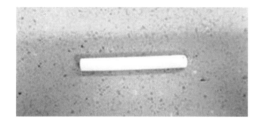

Instrument: High Velocity Saliva Evacuation (HVE)

Function: To evacuate large volumes of fluid and debris from oral cavity

Characteristics: Straight or slightly angled at one or both end; stainless steel, autoclavable plastic, or disposable plastics; attaches to tubing on dental unit

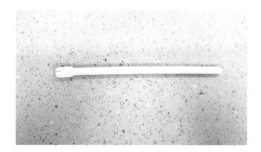

Instrument: Low Velocity saliva evacuation (LVE)

Function: To evacuate reduced volumes of fluid from oral cavity

Characteristics: Disposable plastic for single use; can be bent or used straight; attaches to tubing on dental unit

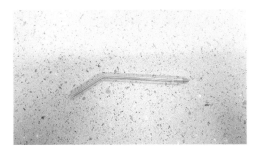

Instrument: Air / Water Syringe Tip

Function: To rinse and dry specific teeth or entire oral cavity

Characteristics: Three-way syringe: air, water, or spray with water and air; Syringe tip; Disposable plastic or autoclavable metal; attaches to air/ water syringe on dental unit

Basic Tray Set- UP

Operative Instruments Amalgam and Composite

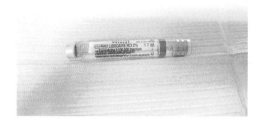

Instrument: Lidocaine- Red

Function: An anesthetic with epinephrine

Characteristics: 2% Lidocaine 1:100,000 epinephrine has a red band on the carpule; most used anesthetic

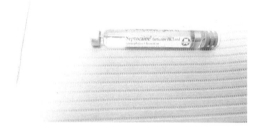

Instrument: Septocaine (articaine HCI and epinephrine)- Gold

Function: An anesthetic with epinephrine

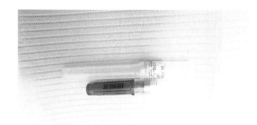

Characteristics: Articaine Hydrochloride 4% and epinephrine 1:100,000

Instrument: Anesthetic Needle

Function: To inject anesthetic into soft tissue

Characteristics: Varies in gauge and length Typically shorts for maxillary typically long for mandibular

Operative Instruments Amalgam and Composite

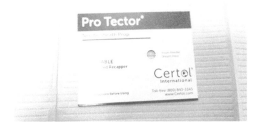

Instrument: Needle stick protector

Function: To hold needle sheath for one- handed recapping after injection, prevent needle stick

Characteristics: Metal and card board protector

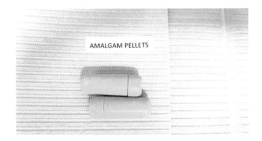

Instrument: Amalgam Capsule

Function: Material used to restore a cavity, build up for crown

Characteristics: contains amalgam, has to be triturated, times differ on types of amalgams

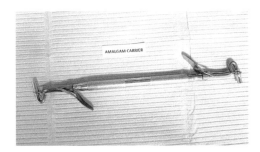

Instrument: Amalgam Carrier

Function: To carry and dispense amalgam for cavity preparation

Characteristics: Amalgam is placed in hollow tubes, and is then placed in cavity preparation, double or single sided

Operative Instruments Amalgam and Composite

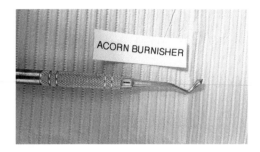

Instrument: Acorn Burnisher

Function: To smooth amalgam after condensing, used to create occlusal anatomy, burnish amalgam

Characteristics: Acorn shaped tip, metal, single or double sided

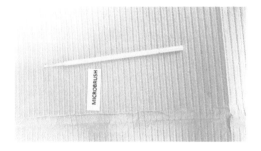

Instrument: Micro Brush

Function: Use to apply primer, dentin bond enamel bond, sealants

Characteristics: Small plastic instrument with small fiber bristled head

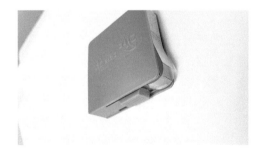

Instrument: Mylar Strip

Function: Thin clear strip used to isolate cavity prep, able to uses light

Characteristics: Similar size to matrix band, clear

Operative Instruments Amalgam and Composite

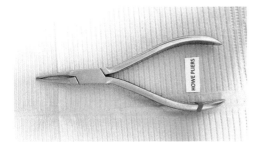

Instrument: Howe Pliers

Function: Also referred to as no pliers. Useful for holing items, for carrying cotton products to and from the oral cavity, removing the matrix band, and placing and removing the wedge

Characteristics: Straight and angulated beaks with serrated tips - specially suited for procedures in the lingual and posterior regions. Essential for insertion and removal of horizontal, vertical, and Wilson (RMO) lingual attachmentss.

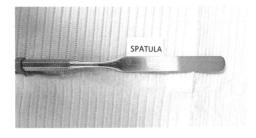

Instrument: Spatulas

Function: Used to mix cements, bases and liners

Characteristics: Straight instrument with flat end for mixing comes in many sizes and shapes

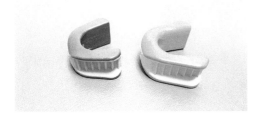

Instrument: Bite Block

Function: Used to prop mouth open for treatment

Characteristics: They come is a variety of sizes and shapes

Operative Instruments Amalgam and Composite

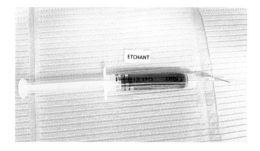

Instrument: Etch

Function: To remove the smear layer, prepare the tooth for bonding

Characteristics: Differs in color and pH level. Concentration of Phosphoric Acid

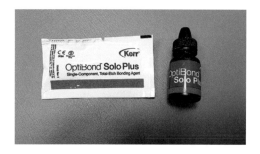

Instrument: Bonding Agents

Function: Acts as an adhesive between the tooth composite material

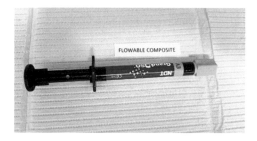

Characteristics: Differs in generation, all in one unit, 3 step, 2 step, brands require different techniques

Instrument: Flowable Composite

Function: High viscosity, low filler composite, used small areas or before placement of packable composite, differs in shade

Characteristics: Fluid like composite, in a syringe used with a syringe tip

Operative Instruments Amalgam and Composite

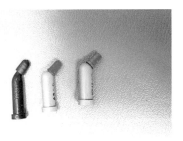

Instrument: Packable Composite

Function: Low viscosity, high filler, permanent restorative material

Characteristics: Either in a syringe or composite tip. Composite tip requires composite gun

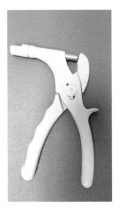

Instrument: Composite Gun

Function: Holds composite tip, used to deliver composite to the cavity preparation

Characteristics: Composite tip inserts in the barrel of the composite gun

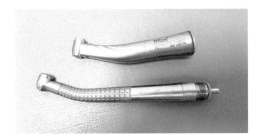

Instrument: High Speed Handpiece

Function: To be used with a bur to cut a cavity/ crown prep

Characteristics: Runs on air pressure, up to 400,000 rpm's, sprays water, friction grip

Operative Instruments Amalgam and Composite

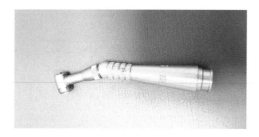

Instrument: Low speed handpiece

Function: To remove decay, polish, open pulpal access, endo refine prep

Characteristics: Runs on air, up to 30,000 rpm's latch and friction grip

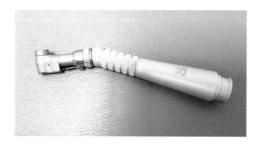

Instrument: Contra Angle

Function: To use with slow speed motor

Characteristics: Different designs for different procedures, hygiene tray, operative tray, surgical tray

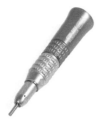

Instrument: Straight nose cone

Function: To use with or without attachments: contra angle or prophy angle; to use with a longshank straight bur

Characteristics: Runs at max 30,000 rpm; use outside oral cavity unless used with attachment

Operative Instruments Amalgam and Composite

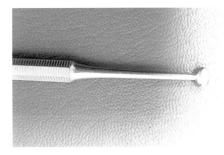

Instrument: Football Burnisher

Function: To smooth Amalgam after condensing, to contour matrix band, to burnish amalgam

Characteristics: Smooth football shaped metal instrument, single or double sided

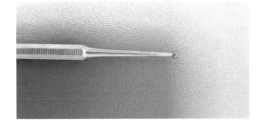

Instrument: Ball Burnisher

Function: to smooth amalgam after condensing to contour matrix band before amalgam placement

Characteristics: Burnishes alloy restorations, single or double sided

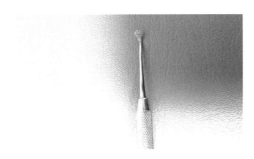

Instrument: Tanner Carver

Function: To carve occlusal anatomy into amalgam restorations

Characteristics: Double ended, ends are shaped to carve alloy restorations, sharp

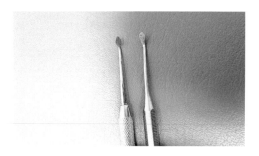

Instrument: Discoid- Cleoid Carver

Function: To carve occusal anatomy into amalgam restorations

Characteristics: Doubaped ended: discoid is disk shaped: cleoid is pointed

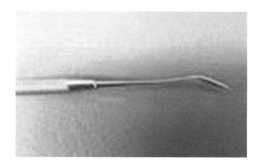

Instrument: Hollenback Carver

Function: To contour and carve occlusal and interproximal anatomy in amalgam restorations

Characteristics: Double ended, sharp stiff metal blade, sharp point; ends are protrude at different angles; carves other restorations materials

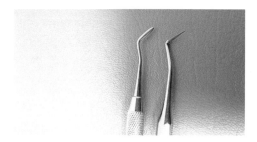

Instrument: Half- Hollenback Carver

Function: To contour and carve occlusal and interproximal anatomy in amalgam restorations

Characteristics: Half the size of Hollenback; Double ended, sharp stiff metal blade, sharp point; ends are protrude at different angles; carves other restorations materials

Operative Instruments Amalgam and Composite

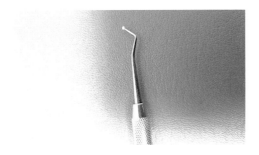

Instrument: Spoon Excavator

Function: To remove carious dentin to remove temp cement, provisional crowns

Characteristics: Spoon- shaped with a cutting edge, small and large sizes

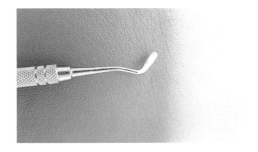

Instrument: Wood Wedges

Function: To hold matrix band in place along gingival margin of class II

Characteristics: Triangular or rounded plastic or wooden, various sizes and color

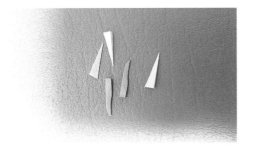

Instrument: Plastic Instrument

Function: To carry composite material for cavity preparation, and shape composite

Characteristics: Specially coated instrument

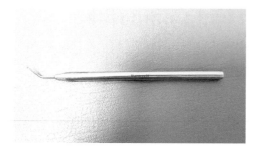

Instrument: Dycal/ Liner Applicator

Function: To Place Calcium Hydroxide or Glass Ionomer

Characteristics: Has short or long handle, similar to a tiny ball burnisher

Operative Instruments Amalgam and Composite

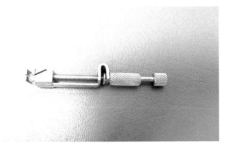

Instrument: Tofflemire/ Matrix Band retainer

Function: To maintain stability of matrix band during condensation of restorations

Characteristics: Has a guide slot, spindle, outer and inner knob

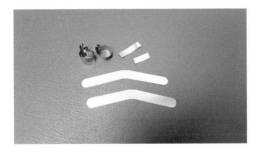

Instrument: Matrix Band

Function: To replace missing proximal walls of cavity preparation for condensation of restorative material

Characteristics: Universal, premolar, molar, and pediatric bands

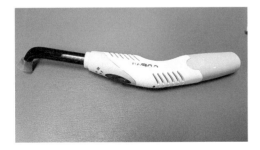

Instrument: Curing Light

Function: To harden light- cure materials, bonding, composites, sealants, cements, build up

Characteristics: Material must be cured in increments of 2mm or less

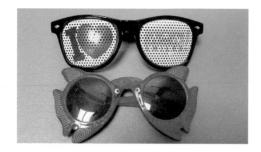

Instrument: Protective Eye Wear

Function: To protect operator' s and assistant's eye during procedures

Characteristics: Orange, dark, clear, protects eyes

Operative Instruments Amalgam and Composite

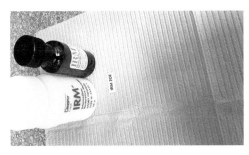 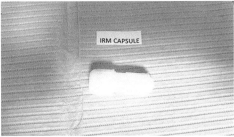

Instrument: IRM (ZOE)

Function: Used as a temporary filling material, sedative filling

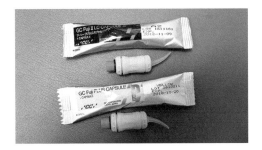

Instrument: Fuji IX or Fuji II

Function: Used for restorative material for high caries risk, releases fluoride

Characteristics: Triturable capsules or liquid powder

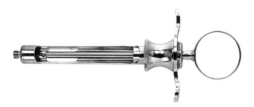

Instrument: Anesthetic Syringe

Function: To administer local anesthetic

Characteristics: Aspirating and self- aspirating syringe. Aspiration syringes have a barb that inserts in the carpule

Operative Instruments Amalgam and Composite

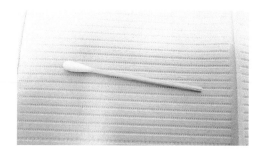

Instrument: Q- Tip

Function: To apply topical anesthetic

Characteristics: Cotton tipped wooden/ plastic stick

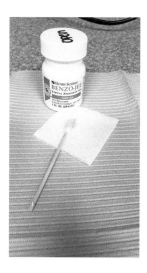

Instrument: Topical Anesthetic

Function: To aid in painless anesthetic

Characteristics: Gel consistency, applied with Q- tip to the injection site, differs in color and taste

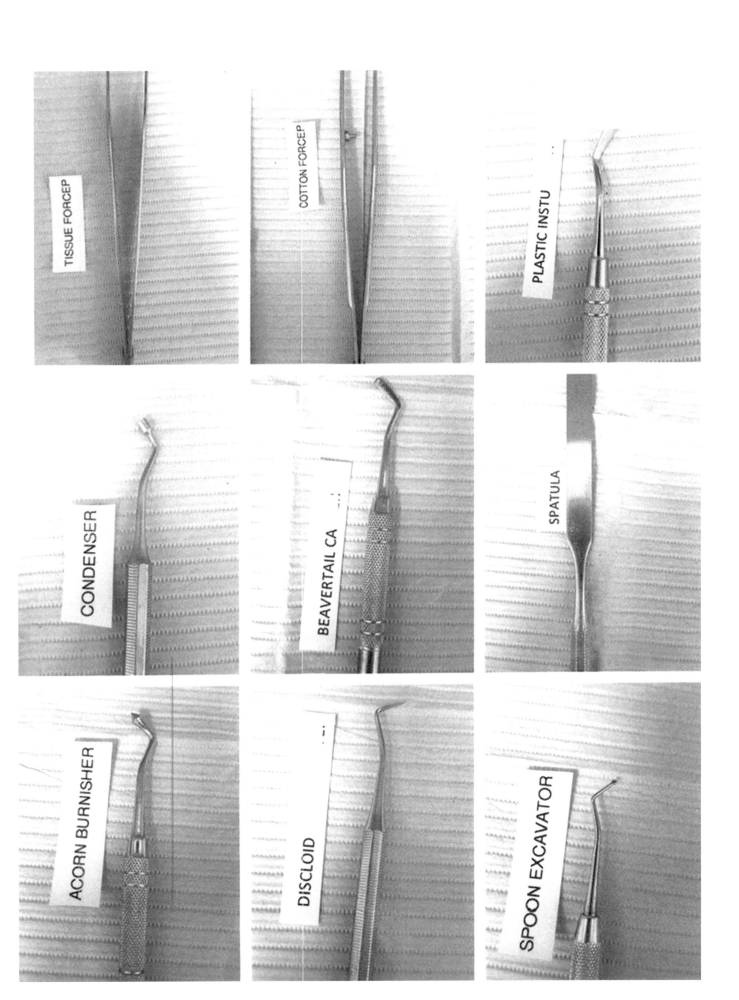

TISSUE FORCEP

COTTON FORCEP

PLASTIC INSTU

CONDENSER

BEAVERTAIL CA

SPATULA

ACORN BURNISHER

DISCLOID

SPOON EXCAVATOR

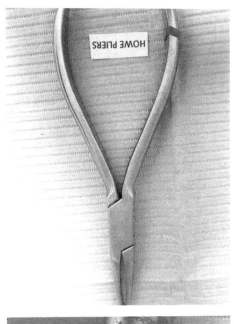

HOWE PLIERS

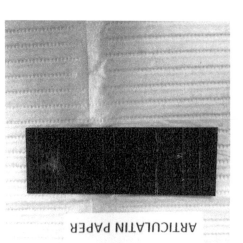

ARTICULATIN PAPER

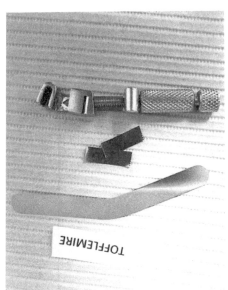

TOFFLEMIRE

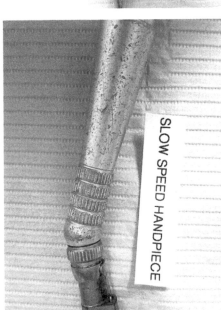

SLOW SPEED HANDPIECE

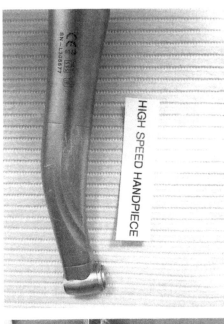

HIGH SPEED HANDPIECE

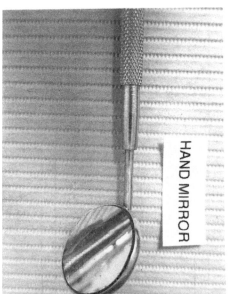

HAND MIRROR

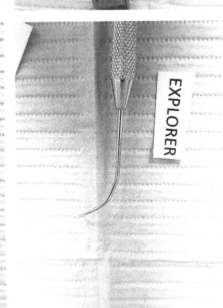

EXPLORER

SICKLE SCALAR

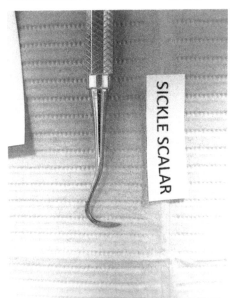

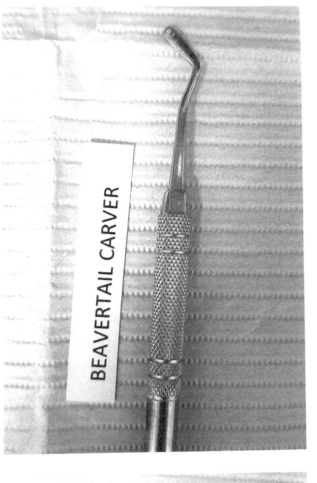

BEAVERTAIL CARVER

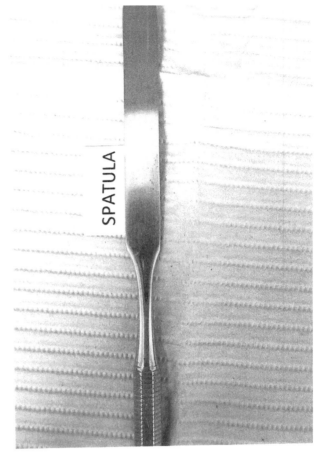

SPATULA

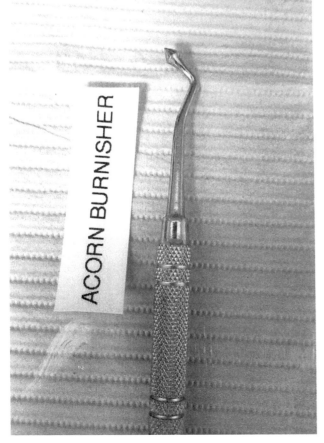

ACORN BURNISHER

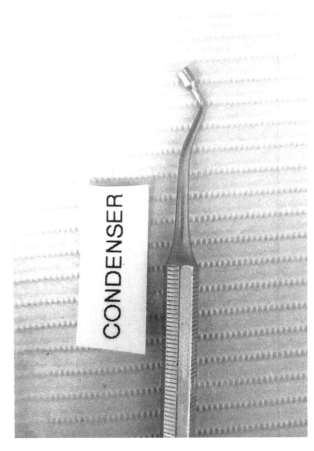

CONDENSER

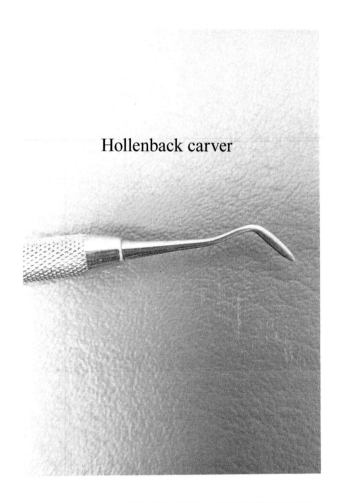

Hollenback carver

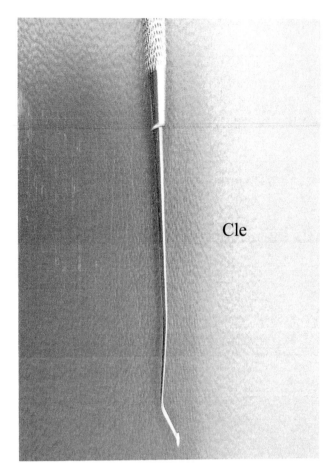

Cle

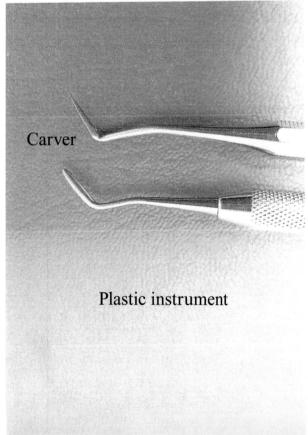

Carver

Plastic instrument

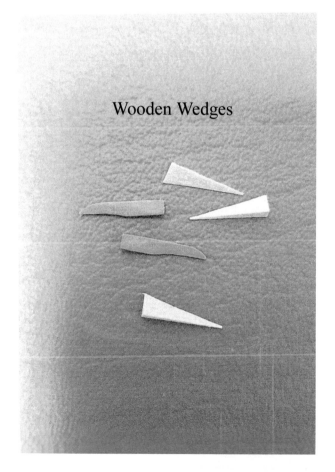

Wooden Wedges

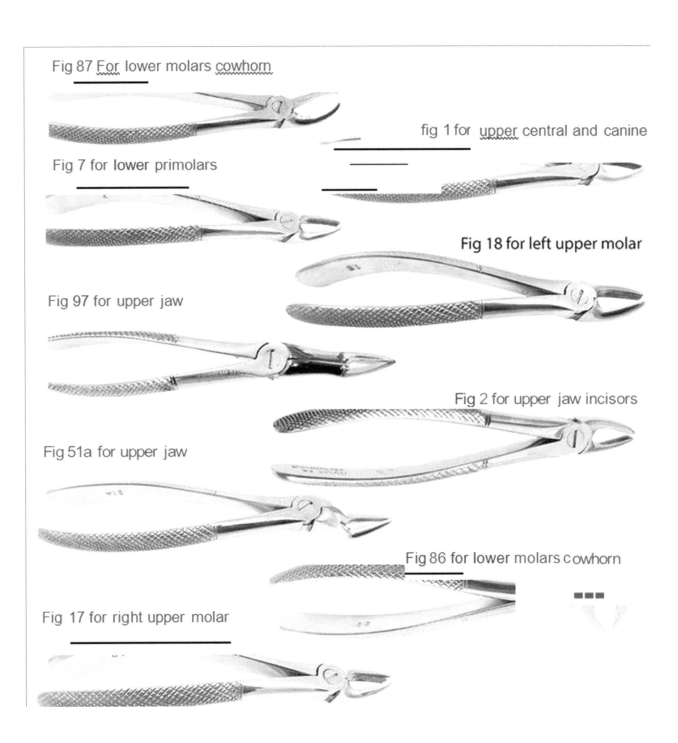

Fig 87 For lower molars cowhorn

fig 1 for upper central and canine

Fig 7 for lower primolars

Fig 18 for left upper molar

Fig 97 for upper jaw

Fig 2 for upper jaw incisors

Fig 51a for upper jaw

Fig 86 for lower molars cowhorn

Fig 17 for right upper molar

Operative Instruments Amalgam and Composite

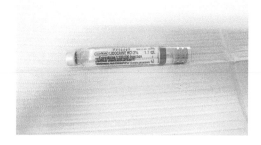

Instrument: Lidocaine- Red

Function: An anesthetic with epinephrine

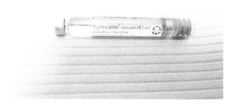

Characteristics: 2% Lidocaine 1:100,000 epinephrine has a red band on the carpule; most used anesthetic

Instrument: Septocaine (articaine HCI and epinephrine)- Gold

Function: An anesthetic with epinephrine

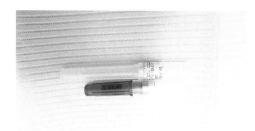

Characteristics: Articaine Hydrochloride 4% and epinephrine 1:100,000

Instrument: Anesthetic Needle

Function: To inject anesthetic into soft tissue

Characteristics: Varies in gauge and length Typically shorts for maxillary typically long for mandibular

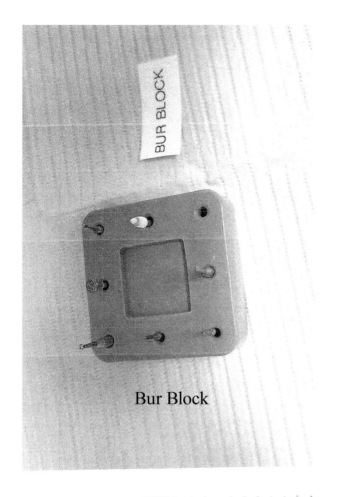

Bur Block

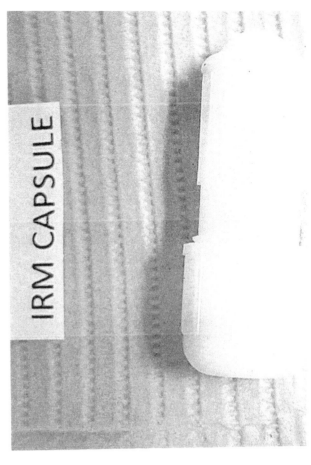

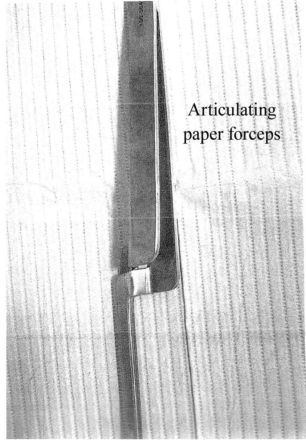

Articulating
paper forceps

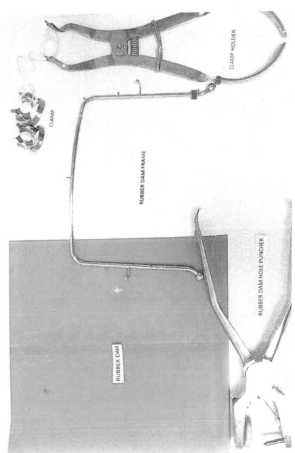

Operative Instruments Amalgam and Composite

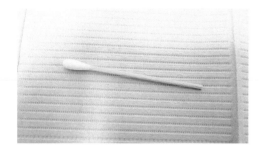

Instrument: Q- Tip

Function: To apply topical anesthetic

Characteristics: Cotton tipped wooden/ plastic stick

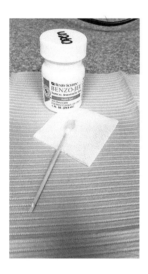

Instrument: Topical Anesthetic

Function: To aid in painless anesthetic

Characteristics: Gel consistency, applied with Q- tip to the injection site, differs in color and taste

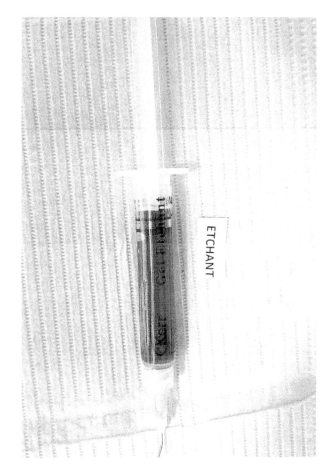

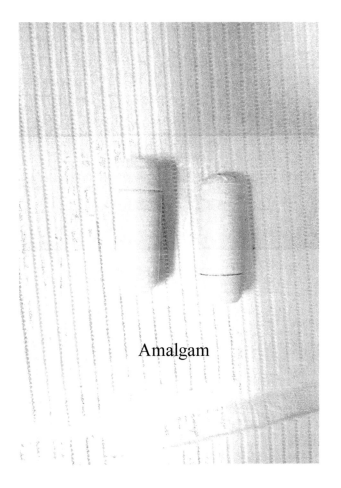

ETCHANT

Amalgam

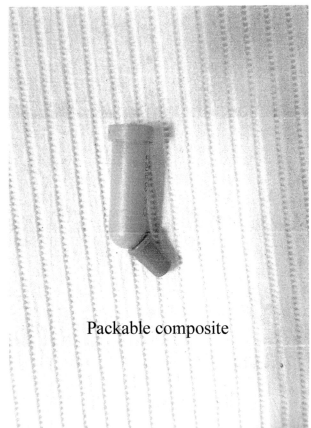

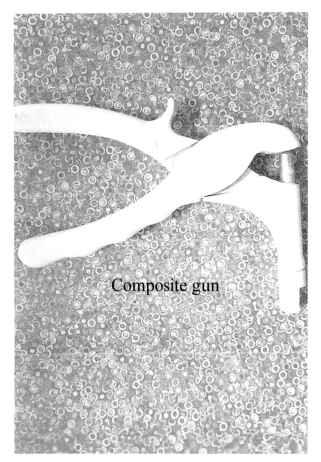

Packable composite

Composite gun

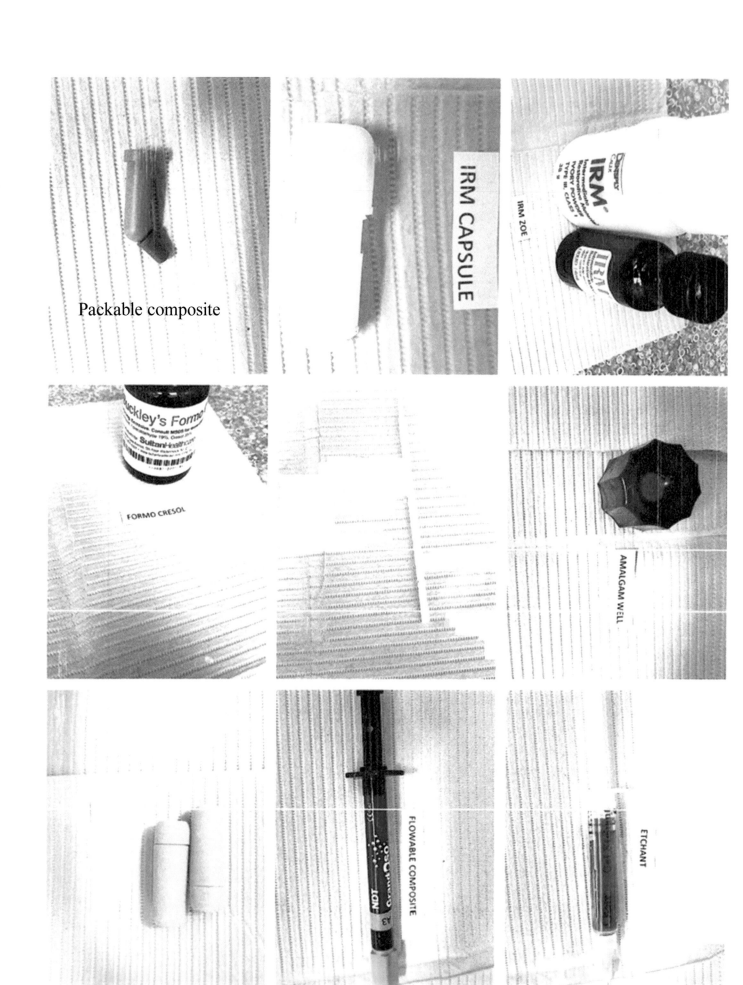

Packable composite

IRM CAPSULE

IRM ZOE

FORMO CRESOL

AMALGAM WELL

FLOWABLE COMPOSITE

ETCHANT

Anesthetic syringe and needle and needle sheath: Prepare Topical anesth and if local anesthesia is required for all treatment trays

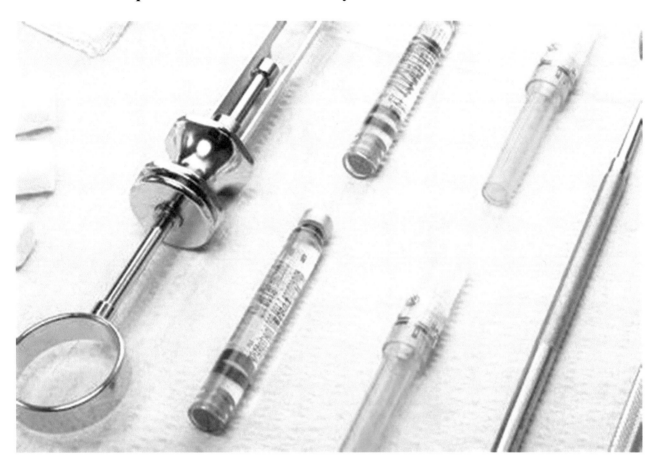

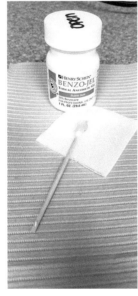

Topical anesthetic

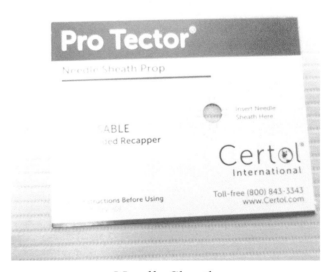

Needle Sheath

Pediatric Stainless Steel Crowns

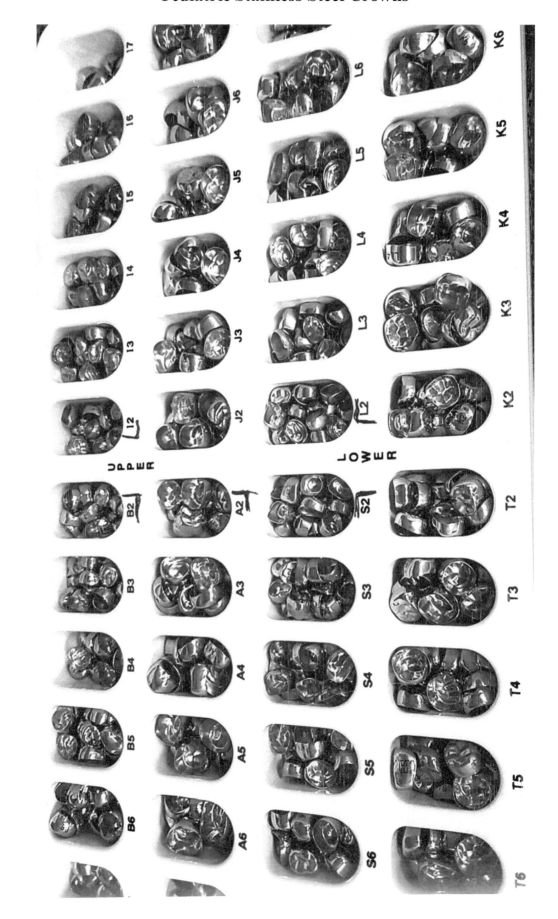

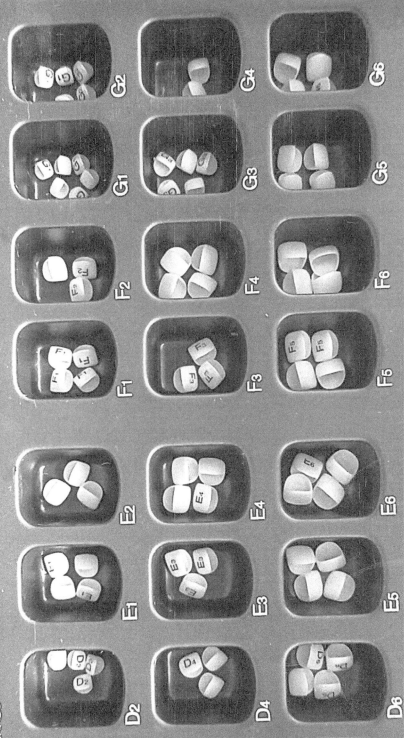

ANTERIOR COLLECTION

Web: www.ezpedo.com • E-mail: info@ezpedo.com • Phone: 888.5.ezpedo

L LATERALS

L CENTRALS

R CENTRALS

R LATERALS

UNIVERSAL LOWER ANTERIORS

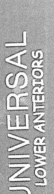
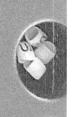

Xrays

The importance of X-ray licensing, a full set of X-rays, what needs to be captured in the X- rays, the indications of infection and decay in X-rays, what a Panoramic X-ray is, how often X- rays are taken for adults and children, and the mandated laws on lead vest and thyroid protection:

X-ray Licensing: In dentistry, X-ray licensing is essential to ensure that dental professionals have the necessary knowledge and skills to operate X-ray equipment safely and effectively. It involves completing specific educational requirements and passing a licensing exam. This licensing is crucial as it ensures patient safety and reduces the risk of radiation exposure.

Full Set of X-rays: A full set of X-rays, also referred to as a "full mouth series," is a comprehensive set of dental X-rays that captures images of all the teeth and surrounding structures. Typically, a full set includes 18 to 20 X-rays, including periapical X-rays, bitewing X-rays, and panoramic X-rays. This comprehensive series provides valuable information about oral health, including areas that may not be visible during a routine examination.

Capturing X-rays: During X-ray taking, it is important to capture specific areas. Apex X-rays are taken to assess the root tips of the teeth, while bitewing X-rays capture the approximal surfaces (contact areas between teeth). These X-rays are crucial in detecting cavities, evaluating bone levels, and assessing the overall oral health of the patient.

Indications in X-rays: X-rays are incredibly useful in diagnosing various conditions in dentistry. They can identify dental decay, bone loss, position and eruption of teeth, root fractures, cysts, and tumors. Additionally, X-rays can reveal signs of infection, such as abscesses or areas of inflammation.

Panoramic X-ray: A Panoramic X-ray is a wide-ranging X-ray that captures the entire upper and lower jaws, providing a broad view of the teeth, jaws, temporomandibular joint, and surrounding structures. This type of X-ray is commonly used to evaluate impacted teeth, assess bone levels, detect tumors or cysts, and aid in treatment planning for orthodontics and oral surgery.

Frequency of X-rays: The frequency of X-rays varies depending on the individual patient's oral health needs. For adults with good oral health, a full set of X-rays is typically taken every 3 to 5 years.

Bitewing X-rays, which are more focused on detecting cavities, are usually taken every 1 to 2 years. For children, X-rays may be taken more frequently to monitor the development of their teeth and detect any orthodontic or dental issues.

Laws on Lead Vest and Thyroid Protection: It is mandated by law to use lead vests and thyroid protection during X-ray procedures. Lead vests are worn by both patients and dental professionals to shield them from unnecessary radiation exposure. Thyroid protection, usually in the form of a thyroid collar, is used to protect the thyroid gland from radiation during X-ray procedures. These safety measures are in place to prioritize the well-being and safety of both patients and dental staff.

Wiggle bug

This is a wiggle bug, also known as an amalgam shaker or amalgamator, is a device commonly found in the dentist office. It is used to mix dental amalgam, which is a filling material used to restore teeth.

The name "wiggle bug" likely comes from the motion of the device as it shakes or vibrates to mix the components of the dental amalgam. The purpose of using an amalgamator is to ensure that the powdered alloy and liquid mercury are thoroughly mixed to create a consistent and smooth amalgam mixture.

The dental amalgam itself is a mixture of powdered metals, such as silver, tin, and copper, combined with liquid mercury. These components are mixed together to create a pliable material that can easily be shaped and placed in a prepared tooth cavity. Once the dental amalgam is placed in the tooth, it hardens and forms a strong, durable filling.

The wiggle bug or amalgam shaker simplifies the amalgam mixing process, ensuring that the alloy and mercury are evenly distributed and properly integrated. This helps to ensure the longevity and effectiveness of the dental restorations placed by the dentist.

Dental cements are commonly used in various dental procedures, such as cementing crowns and bridges, orthodontic bands, and temporary restorations. These cements come in powder and liquid forms that need to be mixed thoroughly to achieve the desired consistency and working time. The wiggle bug can be utilized to shake dental cement capsules, ensuring proper amalgamation of the components before application.

IRM capsules contain intermediate restorative material (IRM), which is a type of temporary filling material used in certain dental situations. The capsules contain a powdered IRM material and a liquid component that need to be mixed together prior to use. The wiggle bug can be used to shake the IRM capsules, ensuring a complete and uniform mixture for effective temporary dental restorations.

It's worth noting that the specific applications of the wiggle bug or amalgam shaker might vary depending on the dental office's preferences and the materials they use. But it is indeed a versatile device commonly used for mixing various dental materials in a consistent and efficient manner.

It is important to note that the use of dental amalgam and amalgamators is a matter of professional decision and choice. There are alternative materials available for dental restorations, such as tooth-colored composites, that do not require the use of amalgam mixers

Wig L Bug

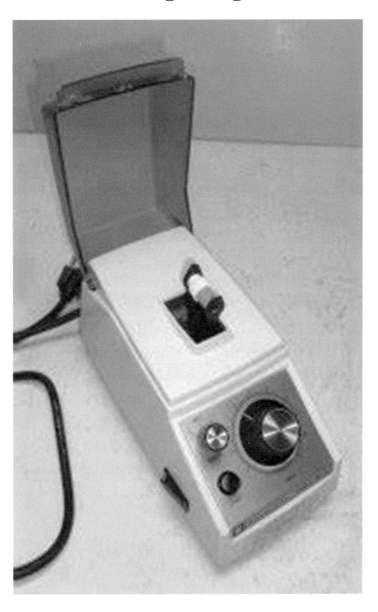

Cure Light

A cure light, also known as a dental curing light or dental curing unit, is a handheld device used in dentistry for polymerizing or hardening dental materials that are light-curable. It emits a specific wavelength of light, typically in the blue range, to activate a photoinitiator within the dental materials and initiate the polymerization process.

The main purpose of a cure light is to cure dental composites, which are tooth-colored resin materials used for filling cavities or restoring teeth. When a composite filling or restoration is placed in a tooth, it is initially soft and malleable. The cure light is then used to shine the light directly onto the composite material, causing it to harden and bond to the tooth structure.

The curing light's emitted light helps initiate a chemical reaction within the composite material, converting it from a soft, pliable state to a hard, durable state. This process is known as polymerization. By curing the composite material, the cure light ensures that the filling or restoration is solidified and capable of withstanding the forces of biting and chewing.

In addition to composite restorations, cure lights can also be used to cure other light-curable dental materials, such as dental sealants, dental adhesives, and certain orthodontic brackets. The versatility and convenience of cure lights make them a standard tool in dental offices for a wide range of restorative and preventive procedures.

It's worth mentioning that dental curing lights come in different designs, with varying light intensities, sizes, and features. Some may have a cord connecting them to a power source, while others may be cordless and rechargeable. The specific type of curing light used can depend on the dentist's preference and the specific needs of the dental practice.

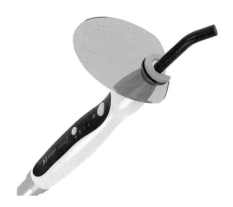

Cavitron

A Cavitron dental tool is an ultrasonic scaler used in dental procedures for both cleaning and treating various dental conditions. It uses ultrasonic vibrations to clean teeth and remove plaque, tartar, and stains from the tooth surface, gum line, and the areas beneath the gum line.

Hygienists and dentists prefer using the Cavitron for several reasons. Firstly, its ultrasonic vibrations create high-frequency sound waves, which help to break down and remove plaque and tartar effectively. This results in a more thorough and efficient cleaning compared to traditional cleaning methods.

Secondly, the Cavitron is more comfortable for patients. The ultrasonic vibrations create tiny bubbles in the water that surrounds the dental tool. These bubbles implode on the tooth surface, providing a gentle and massaging sensation, and reducing discomfort during the procedure.

Moreover, the Cavitron can also be used to perform certain dental treatments, such as root planning and periodontal therapy. It effectively removes calculus and bacteria from the deep pockets between the teeth and gums, leading to improved gum health and reduced risk of gum disease.

Additionally, the Cavitron is versatile and allows the dental professional to adjust the frequency and power settings according to the patient's needs. This customization ensures a tailored treatment plan for each individual.

Overall, the Cavitron dental tool offers advanced technology, improved efficiency, enhanced patient comfort, and effective treatment outcomes, making it a preferred choice for dental cleanings and certain dental treatments by dental professionals.

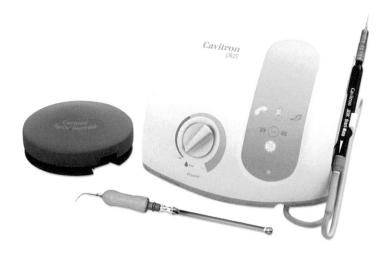

Prophy Tray:

A prophylaxis procedure is performed to remove plaque, tartar (calculus), and stains from the patient's teeth, promoting oral health and preventing gum disease. Here's a breakdown of the typical tools and setup involved:

1. Dental Loupes: The dentist may wear dental loupes with magnification glasses to enhance their vision and precision during the cleaning procedure.

2. Dental Chair: The patient will be seated on the dental chair, which can be adjusted for optimal comfort and access to the oral cavity.

3. Dental Bib and Napkin: A bib and napkin will be placed around the patient's neck to protect their clothing and keep them comfortable during the procedure.

4. Dental Mirror: The dentist will use a dental mirror to aid in visualizing all surfaces of the teeth, including hard-to-reach areas behind or between teeth.

5. Dental Explorer: A dental explorer, a thin, long instrument with a sharp point at one end, is used to detect the presence of cavities, plaque, or tartar buildup.

6. Scalers and Curettes: Scalers and curettes are dental instruments with sharp tips used to remove plaque, tartar, and stains from the tooth surfaces and below the gumline. These instruments may include a variety of shapes and sizes based on the specific tooth surfaces being cleaned.

7. Ultrasonic Scaling Device: An ultrasonic scaler is a handheld instrument that uses high - frequency vibrations to dislodge and remove plaque, tartar, and stains. It is effective for faster and more efficient cleaning, particularly in areas with heavy tartar buildup.

8. Air/Water Syringe: The dental unit will have an air/water syringe to deliver a combination of compressed air and water for rinsing and drying during the dental cleaning procedure.

9. Dental Polishing Handpiece: A dental polishing handpiece, similar to a high -speed handpiece, is used with a prophy cup or brush to apply a polishing paste or pumice to the tooth surfaces.

10. Polishing Paste: A polishing paste, often flavored, is applied to the prophy cup or brush and used to polish the tooth enamel, removing stains and creating a smooth, shiny surface

11. Suction System: A suction system is utilized to remove excess saliva, water, and debris from the patient's mouth during the cleaning procedure, ensuring a clear working field.

12. Dental Floss: Floss may be used to clean between the teeth and below the gumline to remove plaque and debris from tight spaces that scalers and curettes cannot reach.

13. Fluoride Treatment: After the cleaning, the dentist may apply a fluoride gel, rinse, or varnish to strengthen the enamel and provide added protection against cavities.

14. The specific setup and instruments for a prophylaxis dental procedure may vary slightly depending on the dental office and the patient's needs. However, these are the common tools and setup components you can expect to see during a dental cleaning.

Adult Prophy Set Up-

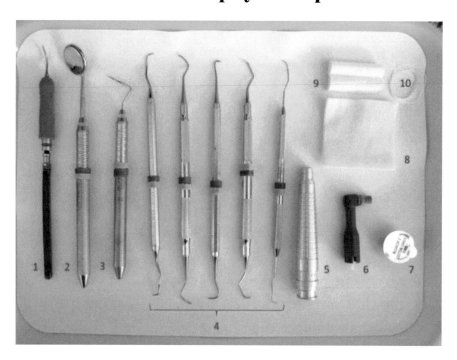

1. Cavitron Tip
2. Mouth mirror
3. Perio Probe
4. Scalers
5. Straight Nose Cone
6. Prophy Angle
7. Prophypast
8. 2X2 Gauze
9. Cotton Rolls
10. **Floss**

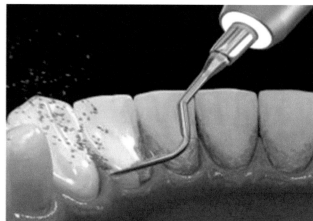

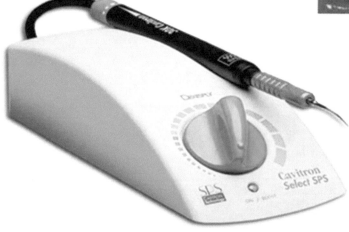

Pediatric prophy set up

1. Mouth mirror
2. Explorer
3. Scalers
4. Straight Nose Cone
5. Prophy Angle
6. Prophy past
7. 2X2 Gauze
8. Floss
9. Saliva Ejector
10. Air water syringe tip

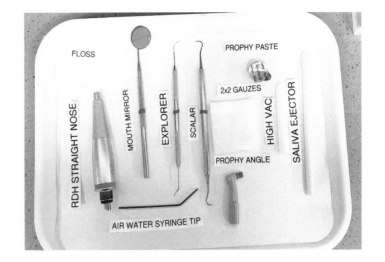

This is how a Cavitron is used

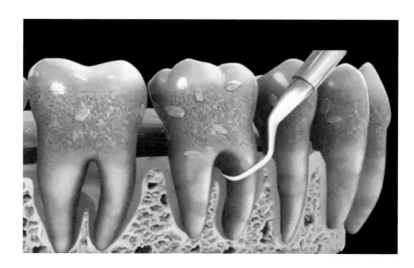

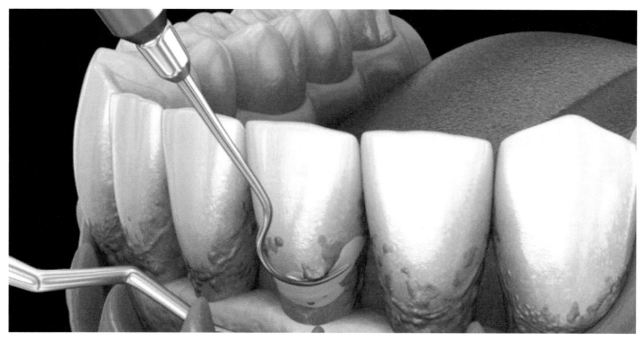

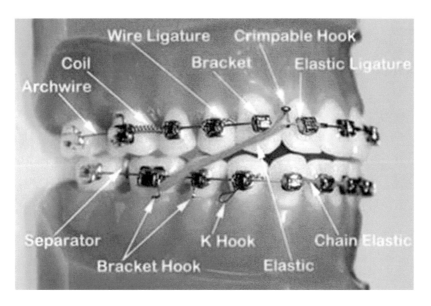

Coil
Archwire
Wire Ligature
Bracket
Crimpable Hook
Elastic Ligature
Separator
Bracket Hook
K Hook
Elastic
Chain Elastic

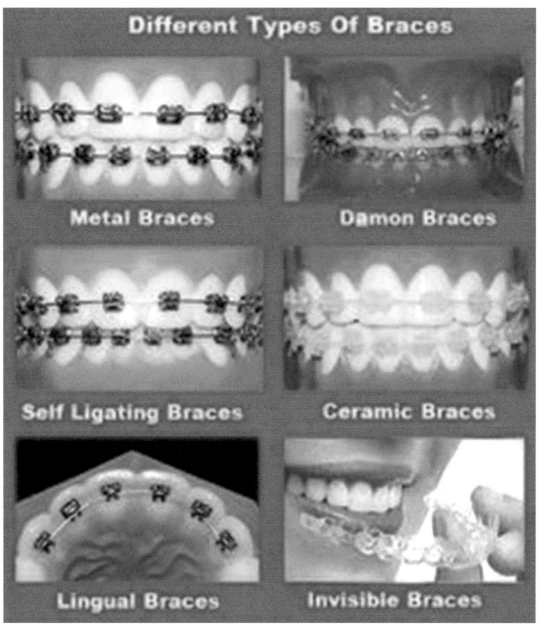

Different Types Of Braces

Metal Braces

Damon Braces

Self Ligating Braces

Ceramic Braces

Lingual Braces

Invisible Braces

Orthodontic

Orthodontics: Dental Assistant Jobs and Duties

Orthodontics is a specialized field in dentistry that focuses on correcting tooth and jaw misalignments. Within this field, dental assistants play a crucial role in supporting orthodontists during various procedures. This article will explore the job responsibilities and duties of dental assistants in orthodontics, with a particular emphasis on tasks such as removing arch wires, ties, taking impressions, and removing orthodontic spacers.

Dental Assistant: An Essential Role in Orthodontics:

A dental assistant is a valuable member of the orthodontic team, responsible for assisting orthodontists in providing patient care. Their duties encompass a wide range of tasks, ensuring the smooth functioning of orthodontic procedures and treatments.

1. Removing Arch Wires:

One of the important duties of a dental assistant is to assist in removing archwires. Archwires are wires that connect brackets, applying gentle pressure to move teeth into their proper position. Dental assistants work closely with orthodontists to carefully remove these wires using specialized tools, ensuring patient comfort and safety.

2. Removing Ties:

Another crucial duty of a dental assistant in orthodontics is removing ties. Ties are small rubber bands that are used to hold archwires in place on the brackets. Dental assistants have the responsibility to carefully remove ties without causing any discomfort or damaging the brackets.

3. Taking Impressions:

Dental assistants are often responsible for taking impressions of patients' teeth. Impressions are used to create models and molds for various orthodontic appliances such as retainers or braces. Assistants must ensure the accuracy of impressions, as they serve as a vital tool for orthodontists to develop customized treatment plans.

4. Removing Orthodontic Spacers:

Orthodontic spacers, also known as separators, are small rubber bands or metal appliances placed between the teeth to create space for orthodontic procedures. Dental assistants play a significant role in removing these spacers by carefully dislodging them using specialized tools. This task requires precision and attention to detail to avoid any discomfort or injury to the patient.

In the realm of orthodontics, dental assistants hold a crucial position in the day-to-day operations of a dental practice. Their roles encompass various tasks, including removing archwires, ties, taking impressions, and removing orthodontic spacers. By efficiently performing these duties, dental assistants contribute to the success of orthodontic treatments and ensure the comfort and satisfaction of patients.

Dental impressions

Dental Impressions are molds or imprints of a patient's teeth, gums, and surrounding oral structures. They are used by dentists to create accurate replicas of a patient's mouth, which are essential for various dental procedures. Impressions serve several purposes, including:

1. Diagnosis: Dentists use impressions to study a patient's oral condition, identify dental issues, and plan appropriate treatment.

2. Prosthodontics: Impressions are crucial for designing and creating dental prosthetics like crowns, bridges, dentures, and dental implants. They help in achieving a precise fit and natural appearance.

3. Orthodontics: Orthodontic treatments, such as braces and aligners, require impressions to assess the current position of the teeth and plan the movement necessary to achieve proper alignment.

4. Restorative Dentistry: Dental impressions help in fabricating restorations like inlays, onlays, and veneers, which are used to repair damaged or decayed teeth.

5. Bite Guards and Splints: Impressions are used to create custom-made bite guards and splints, which provide protection and support for patients with conditions like bruxism (teeth grinding) or temporomandibular joint disorders (TMJ).

Overall, dental impressions play a vital role in accurate diagnosis, treatment planning, and the creation of various dental appliances, ensuring optimal oral health and function for patients.

Aliginate Impression Tray Set- up

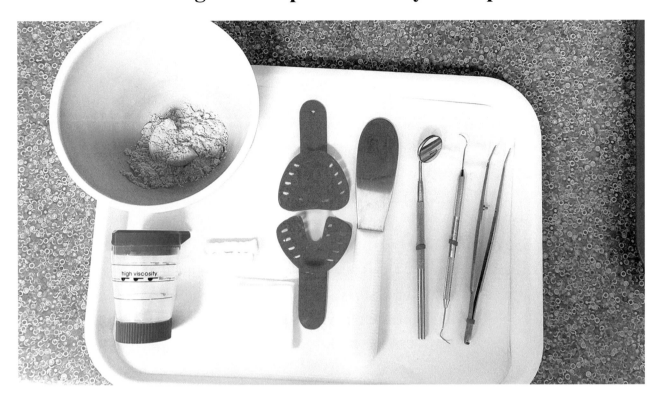

Tray Set- up Instrument

1. **Mixing Bowl**
2. **Alignate Material**
3. **2X2 Gauzes**
4. **Cotton Rolls**
5. **Mixing Spatula**
6. **Lower/ upper impression trays**
7. **Cotton Forcep**
8. **Explorer**
9. **Mouth Mirror**

Composite Filling Instruments:

1. Mouth mirror: Used for providing visibility and reflecting light into the oral cavity.
2. Explorer: Typically a sharp, pointed instrument used for detecting and examining tooth surfaces.
3. Cotton Forceps: Used for holding and manipulating cotton rolls, gauze, or other materials.
4. Spoon Excavator: Used for removing soft carious dentin and debris from the cavity preparation.
5. Hatchet: A cutting instrument with a sharp blade, used for enamel and dentin preparation.
6. Chisel: Used for precise removal of enamel and dentin during the cavity preparation.
7. Gingival Margin Trimmer: Designed to refine the cavosurface margin and create a smooth transition from the restoration to the tooth structure.
8. Composite Placement Instrument: Various types, such as composite carriers, condensers, and burnishers, used for placing, shaping, and compacting the composite material.
9. Composite Carver: Helps to sculpt and contour the composite material to fit the tooth anatomy.
10. Composite Polishing Disk: Used for final polishing of the restoration to achieve a smooth and natural appearance.
11. Articulating Paper Holder with Articulating Paper: Essential for checking the occlusion and adjusting the restoration if necessary.
12. High-speed Handpiece: Typically used with diamond or carbide burs for tooth preparation.
13. Low-speed Handpiece: Used for finishing and polishing the restoration with various attachments such as polishers and brushes.

Tray Setup for Composite Fillings:

1. Dental tray: Choose a suitable tray to organize and hold the instruments and materials.
2. High-speed Handpiece: Place in tray, ensuring it is properly sterilized and ready for use.
3. Low-speed Handpiece: Place in tray alongside the high-speed handpiece.
4. Mouth mirror: Sterilize and place in the tray.
5. Explorer: Sterilize and place in the tray.
6. Cotton forceps: Sterilize and place in the tray.

7. Spoon excavator: Sterilize and place in the tray.
8. Hatchet: Sterilize and place in the tray.
9. Chisel: Sterilize and place in the tray.
10. Gingival margin trimmer: Sterilize and place in the tray.
11. Composite placement instruments: Sterilize and place in the tray.
12. Composite carver: Sterilize and place in the tray.
13. Composite polishing disk: Sterilize and place in the tray.
14. Articulating paper holder with articulating paper: Sterilize and place in the tray.
15. Mixing pad or dappen dish: Use for mixing the composite material.
16. Etchant and bonding agent: Arrange the necessary materials for bonding the composite to the tooth structure.
17. Composite materials: Place various shades and types of composite resin in the tray.
18. Cotton rolls and gauze: Include enough for moisture control during the procedure.
19. Dental dam and dental dam clamp (if applicable): Set up if isolation is required for the procedure.
20. Tooth isolation material: Include materials such as cotton pellets or wedges for isolating the working area.
21. Anesthetic syringe and needle: Prepare if local anesthesia is required.

Composite Filling Instruments:

Composite Tray set-up

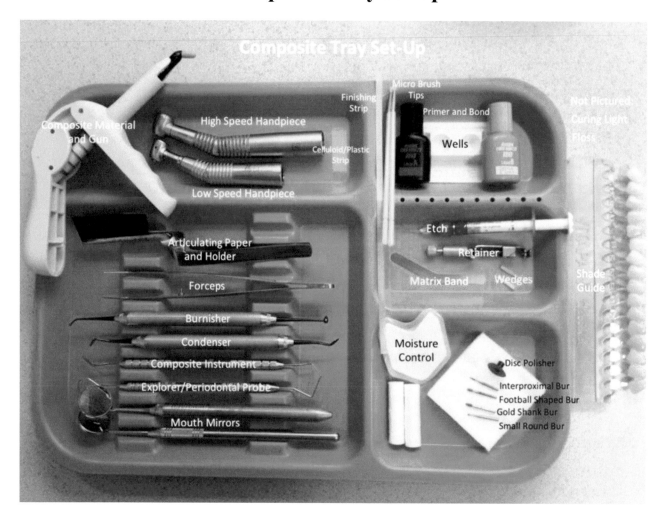

Tray Setup for Composite Fillings:

1. Dental tray: Choose a suitable tray to organize and hold the instruments and materials.
2. High-speed Handpiece: Place in tray, ensuring it is properly sterilized and ready for use.
3. Low-speed Handpiece: Place in tray alongside the high-speed handpiece.
4. Mouth mirror: Sterilize and place in the tray.
5. Explorer: Sterilize and place in the tray.
6. Cotton forceps: Sterilize and place in the tray.
7. Spoon excavator: Sterilize and place in the tray.
8. Hatchet: Sterilize and place in the tray.
9. Chisel: Sterilize and place in the tray.

10. Gingival margin trimmer: Sterilize and place in the tray.

11. Composite placement instruments: Sterilize and place in the tray.

12. Composite carver: Sterilize and place in the tray.

13. Composite polishing disk: Sterilize and place in the tray.

14. Articulating paper holder with articulating paper: Sterilize and place in the tray.

15. Mixing pad or dappen dish: Use for mixing the composite material.

16. Etchant and bonding agent: Arrange the necessary materials for bonding the composite to the tooth structure.

17. Composite materials: Place various shades and types of composite resin in the tray.

18. Cotton rolls and gauze: Include enough for moisture control during the procedure.

19. Dental dam and dental dam clamp (if applicable): Set up if isolation is required for the procedure.

20. Tooth isolation material: Include materials such as cotton pellets or wedges for isolating the working area.

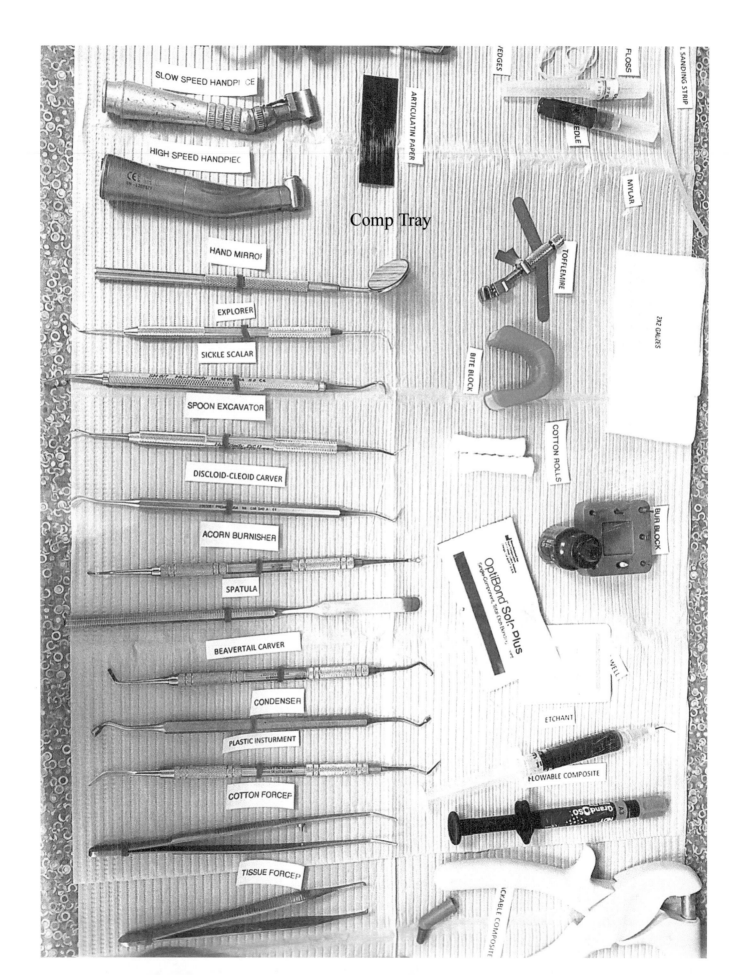

Comp Tray

SLOW SPEED HANDPIECE

HIGH SPEED HANDPIECE

ARTICULATIN PAPER

WEDGES

NEEDLE

FLOSS

L SANDING STRIP

MYLAR

HAND MIRROR

TOFFLEMIRE

EXPLORER

SICKLE SCALAR

BITE BLOCK

2X2 GAUZES

SPOON EXCAVATOR

DISCLOID-CLEOID CARVER

COTTON ROLLS

ACORN BURNISHER

BUR BLOCK

OptiBond Solo Plus
Single-Component Total-Etch Bonding Ad

SPATULA

WELL

BEAVERTAIL CARVER

ETCHANT

CONDENSER

FLOWABLE COMPOSITE

PLASTIC INSTURMENT

GrandioSo A3

COTTON FORCEP

TISSUE FORCEP

CKABLE COMPOSITE

These instruments and tray setup items provide a comprehensive setup for an amalgam filling procedure. Remember to follow your clinician's instructions and refer to the specific requirements of your dental office.

Amalgam

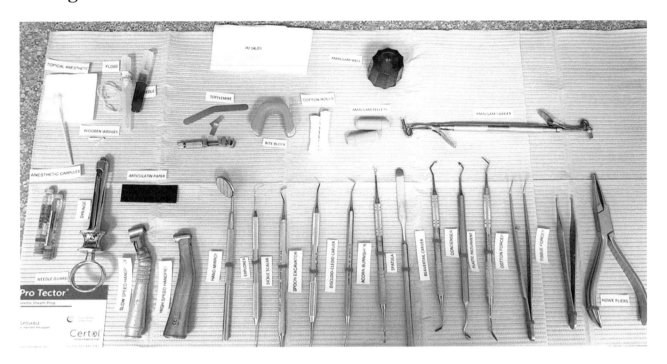

Instruments for Amalgam Filling:

1. Mouth mirror: Used for intraoral examination and tissue retraction.
2. Explorer: A diagnostic instrument used to detect caries and evaluate tooth surfaces.
3. Cotton forceps: Used for placing and removing cotton rolls.
4. High-speed handpiece: Used for initial tooth preparation and removal of decay.
5. Slow-speed handpiece with straight handpiece attachment: Used for finishing and polishing the restoration.
6. Amalgam carrier: Used for carrying and dispensing amalgam into the prepared tooth.
7. Condenser: Used for packing and condensing amalgam into the preparation.
8. Carver (discoid-cleoid or Hollenback): Used for carving and shaping the amalgam restoration.
9. Burnisher: Used for smoothing and shaping the amalgam.
10. Matrix band and retainer: Used to create a tight proximal contact and contour.
11. Wooden wedges: Used to stabilize the matrix band and create a tight contact.
12. Articulating paper: Used for checking occlusion after restoration placement.
13. Floss: Used for finalizing proximal contacts.

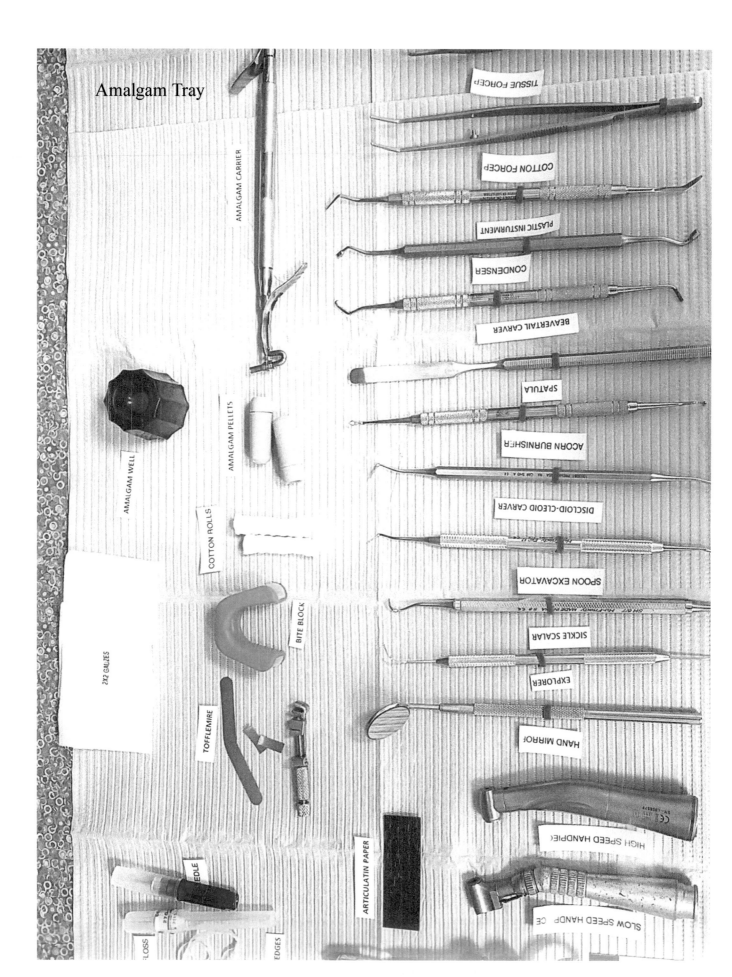

Amalgam Tray

Root Canal Tray:

A root canal tray setup includes specific instruments and materials necessary for a root canal treatment, which involves removing infected pulp from the tooth's root canal system and sealing it to prevent further infection. Here is a breakdown of the typical setup and everything that may be needed:

1. Dental Loupes: The dentist may wear dental loupes with magnification glasses to enhance their vision and precision during the root canal procedure.
2. Dental Chair: The patient will be seated on the dental chair, which can be adjusted for optimal access and comfort during the treatment.
3. Dental Bib and Napkin: A bib and napkin will be placed around the patient's neck to protect their clothing and maintain their comfort during the procedure. Dental Dam: A dental dam is a thin, flexible sheet made of latex or non-latex material. It is used to isolate the tooth being treated, preventing contamination from saliva and allowing better visibility and control during the procedure.
4. Dental Dam Clamp and Forceps: Dental dam clamps are used to secure the dental dam in place around the tooth. They come in different shapes and sizes to fit different teeth. Dental dam forceps are used for placement and removal of the clamps.
5. Dental Dam Punch: A dental dam punch is a specialized instrument used to create precise holes in the dental dam for exposing the tooth being treated and its neighboring teeth.
6. Endodontic Files and Reamers: These fine, flexible instruments are used for cleaning and shaping the root canal. They come in various sizes and shapes, such as K-files and Flex files, and are used sequentially to remove infected pulp and shape the canal for filling.
7. Gates-Glidden Drills: These drills are used to enlarge the access cavity and remove the bulk of the infected pulp from the pulp chamber efficiently.
8. Root Canal Sealers and Medicaments: Various medicaments and root canal sealers, such as calcium hydroxide or resin-based sealers, may be used to irrigate, disinfect, and fill the root canal system after cleaning.
9. Gutta-Percha Points and Obturators: Gutta-percha is a rubber-like material used to fill and seal the root canal after cleaning. Gutta-percha points of different sizes and tapers are selected, and obturators may be used for delivering and compacting the gutta-percha within the canal.

10. Rubber Dam Clamp Forceps: These specialized forceps are used for placement and removal of rubber dam clamps. They aid in securing the rubber dam and maintaining isolation during the procedure.

11. Root Canal Obturation Devices: These devices, such as heated instruments or vertical compaction devices, may be used to condense and seal the gutta-percha within the root canal.

12. Irrigation Solutions and Needles: Various irrigation solutions, such as sodium hypochlorite (bleach) or chlorhexidine, are used to disinfect and irrigate the root canal system. Irrigation needles and syringes are used to deliver these solutions.

13. Paper Points and Absorbent Points: These sterile, absorbent points are used to dry and remove excess fluids from the root canal during the treatment process.

14. Finishing strips: Used for interproximal reduction and contouring.

15. Dental syringe: Used for irrigation and drying of the preparation

16. Apex Locator and Radiograph Devices: These devices are used to measure the length of the root canal accurately and obtain radiographic images for guidance during the procedure..

Endo Tray Set Up

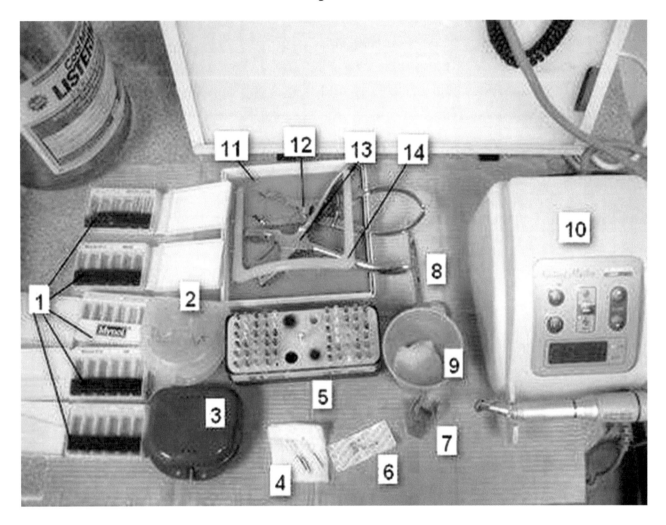

Endodontic Therapy (Part 1) –

Instruments Required by the root canal specialist:

1. Gutta Percha Points (Various Sizes)
2. Rubber Dam Clamps (Molars)
3. Rubber Dam Clamps (Anterior)
4. Peeso Reamers (Sizes 1, 2 and 3)
5. Endodontic Files Organizer (21mm and 25mm)
6. Carbide Bur
7. Thumb Ruler
8. Curved Scissors
9. Soaked Cotton 2×2 (Isopropyl Alcohol)

10. Endodontic Drill
11. Dental Dam
12. Dental Dam Forceps
13. Dental Dam Punch
14. Dental Dam Frame May Also Require:
15. Apex Locator and Radiograph Devices: These devices are used to measure the length of the root canal accurately and obtain radiographic images for guidance during the procedure.

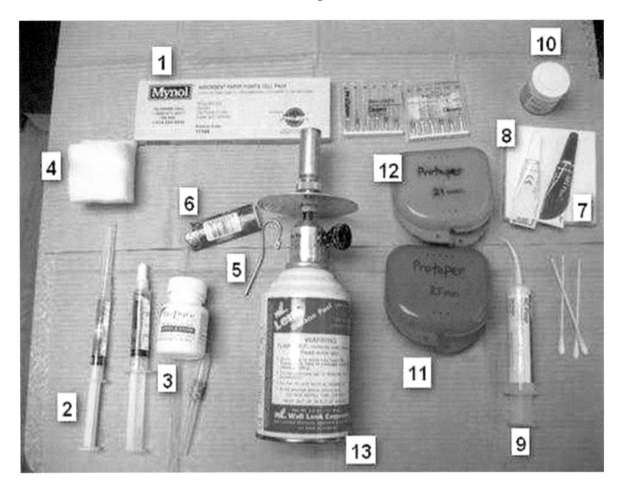

Endodontic Therapy (Part 2) –

Instruments Required by the root canal specialist:

1. Adsorbent Paper Points
2. Sodium Hypochlorite (Syringe and Tip)
3. Bio Pure (Syringe and Powder with Tip)
4. Basic Materials
5. Apex Locator Tip
6. Lighter
7. AH Plus Canal Sealer
8. Mixing Pad
9. RC Prep Syringe
10. Cavit-G Temporary Material
11. Protaper Case (25mm)
12. Protaper Case (21mm)
13. Butane Burner

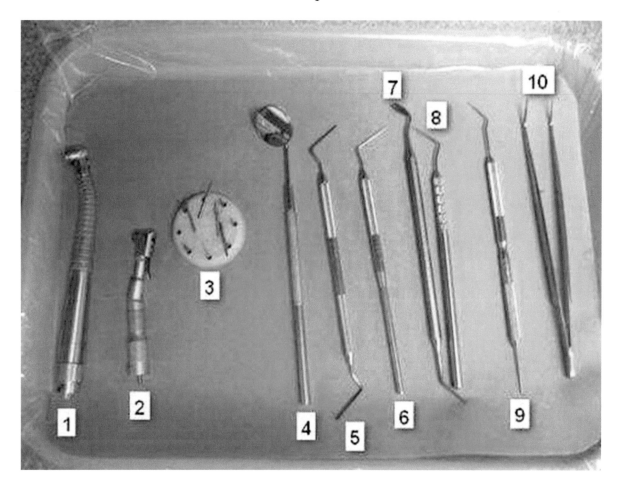

Endodontic Therapy (Part 3) –

Instruments Required by the root canal specialist:

1. High-Speed Drill
2. Slow Speed Attachment
3. Bonding Bur Block
4. Mirror
5. Root Canal Plugger (9-11)
6. Root Canal Plugger (3-5)
7. Glick Carver
8. Spreader (11-21)
9. Explorer – Anterior
10. College PliersMay Also Require:
    1. Slow Speed Drill
    2. Root ZX (Apex Locator)
    3. X-ray Film and XCP (Correspond to Specific Tooth)

Pulpotomy For Primary (Baby Teeth)

A pulpotomy is a dental procedure that involves the removal of the inflamed or infected pulp tissue from the crown portion of a tooth, while preserving the healthy root portion. It is typically performed on primary (baby) teeth to treat extensive decay or dental trauma, and is aimed at saving the tooth and preventing the spread of infection.

Here's a general outline of the steps involved in a pulpotomy procedure:

1. Evaluation and anesthesia: The dentist will examine the tooth and evaluate the extent of decay or injury. Local anesthesia is typically administered to numb the area and ensure patient comfort throughout the procedure.
2. Isolation: The affected tooth is isolated using a dental dam or a specialized clamp to keep it clean and prevent contamination from saliva.
3. Removal of decay: The dentist will access the pulp chamber by creating a small opening in the top of the tooth. Any decayed or infected tissue is carefully removed using dental instruments or a high-speed handpiece.
4. Pulpotomy: After removing the affected pulp tissue, a medicament such as formocresol or mineral trioxide aggregate (MTA) is applied to the remaining healthy pulp tissue to protect and preserve it. The medication helps in disinfecting the area and promoting healing.
5. Restoration: The tooth is then filled with a suitable material, such as a dental composite or stainless-steel crown, to restore its structure, strength, and functionality.
6. Follow-up care: After the pulpotomy, a follow-up appointment may be scheduled to monitor the healing process and ensure there are no complications.

It's important to note that the specific procedures and materials used during a pulpotomy may vary depending on the individual case and the dentist's preference. If you suspect your child needs a pulpotomy or have further questions, it is advisable to consult with a qualified dentist who can provide an accurate diagnosis and personalized treatment plan

Pulpotomy/ Open and Drain

1. Mouth Mirror
2. Endo Explorer
3. Rubber Dam
4. Rubber Dam Clamps
5. Topical
6. Endofiles
7. Cotton Forcep
8. Ruler (to measure files)
9. Articulating paper Holder
10. Articulating paper
11. Floss
12. Cotton Rolls
13. 2X2 Gauzes
14. High Speed Handpiece
15. Bur Block
16. Syringe
17. Anesthetic
18. Needle
19. Sodium Hyporide (Bleach)
20. Broaches
21. Paper Points
22. Calcium Hydroxide
23. IRM
24. Formocresol (Posterior teeth)
25. Cotton Pellets

Pulpotomy Set- Up

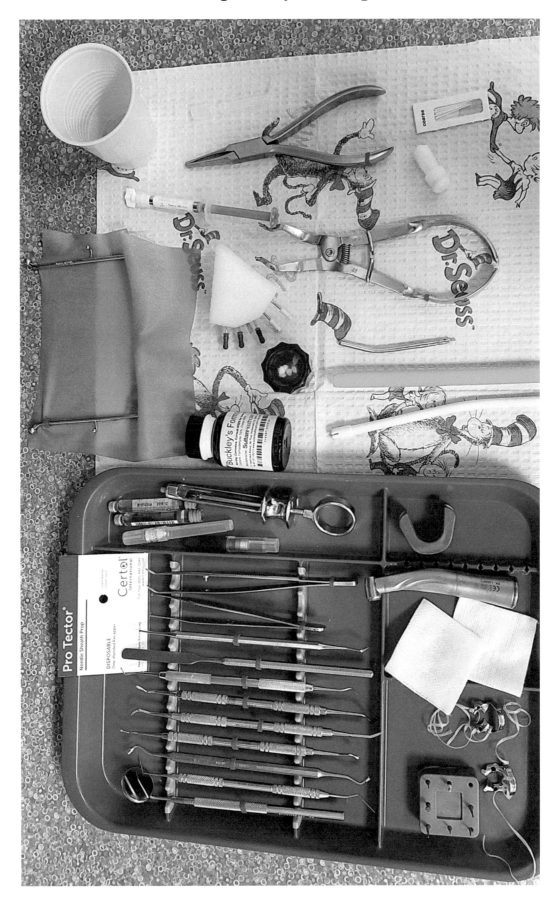

CROWN PREPARATION Tray Setup:

Let's discuss the setup and procedure for an adult crown prep (crown preparation) as well as a pediatric crown prep (crown preparation) separately:

Adult Crown Prep (Crown Preparation):

1. Dental Loupes: The dentist may wear dental loupes with magnification glasses for improved precision and visibility during the crown preparation.

2. Dental Chair: The patient will be seated on the dental chair, which can be adjusted for optimal access and comfort during the procedure.

3. Dental Bib and Napkin: A bib and napkin will be placed around the patient's neck to protect their clothing and maintain their comfort during the procedure.

4. Dental Anesthesia: Local anesthetic will be administered to numb the tooth and surrounding tissues to ensure a pain-free experience for the patient.

5. Dental Dam (Optional): Depending on the dentist's preference and the case, a dental dam may be placed to isolate the tooth being treated. This helps maintain a clean and dry operating field.

6. Dental Handpiece: A high-speed dental handpiece fitted with a diamond or carbide bur is used to remove the decayed or damaged tooth structure and prepare the tooth for the crown.

7. Dental Burs: Various dental burs of different sizes and shapes are used for different stages of crown preparation, including initial tooth reduction, margin refinement, and tooth shaping.

8. Dental Matrix (Optional): In some cases, a dental matrix may be used to create a temporary shape around the prepared tooth to aid in impression-making and temporary crown fabrication.

9. Retraction Cord: A retraction cord may be placed around the gingival margin to gently push back the gum tissue, providing better access and visibility during the procedure.

10. Dental Impression Materials: An impression material, such as polyvinyl siloxane (PVS) or polyether, is used to take an accurate impression of the prepared tooth.

This impression is sent to the dental laboratory for fabrication of the permanent crown.

11. Temporary Crown Material: A temporary crown material, such as acrylic or composite, is used to fabricate a temporary crown that will protect the prepared tooth until the permanent crown is placed.

Crown Prep Tray Set-Up

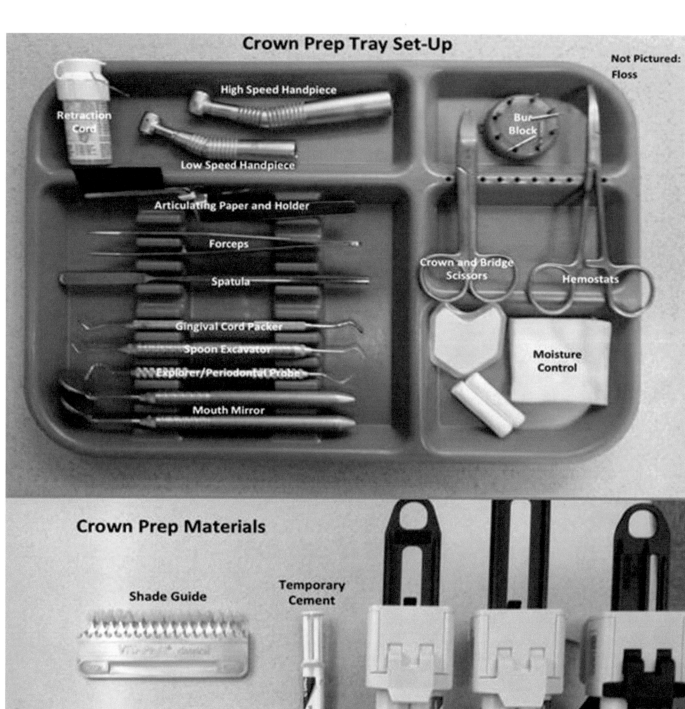

Not Pictured: Floss

Retraction Cord

High Speed Handpiece

Low Speed Handpiece

Bur Block

Articulating Paper and Holder

Forceps

Spatula

Gingival Cord Packer

Spoon Excavator

Explorer/Periodontal Probe

Mouth Mirror

Crown and Bridge Scissors

Hemostats

Moisture Control

Crown Prep Materials

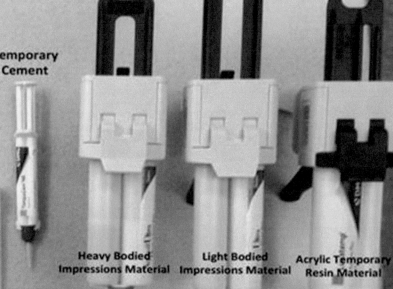

Shade Guide

Temporary Cement

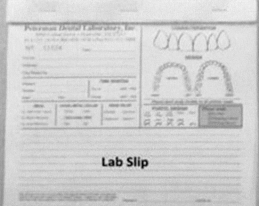

Lab Slip

Heavy Bodied Impressions Material

Light Bodied Impressions Material

Acrylic Temporary Resin Material

Heavy Bodied Mixing Tip

Light Bodied Mixing Tip (Intraoral)

Temporary Resin Mixing Tip

Pediatric Crown Prep (Crown Preparation):

The tools and materials used for pediatric crown preparations are generally similar to those used for adult crown preps. However, there may be some differences due to the unique requirements of treating primary (baby) teeth. Here are a few key differences:

1. Pediatric Restorative Kit: A pediatric restorative kit may contain specialized instruments and smaller-sized burs suitable for the smaller anatomy of primary teeth.

2. Behavior Management Techniques: Pediatric dentists often employ behavior management techniques, such as tell-show-do, positive reinforcement, or sedation, to help children feel comfortable and cooperative during the procedure.

3. Stainless Steel Crowns or pre form porslen white crowns: Instead of tooth-colored porcelain or zirconia crowns used for adult teeth, stainless steel crowns are commonly used in pediatric dentistry due to their durability, cost-effectiveness, and ease of placement.

4. Pediatric-Sized Dental Dam (Optional): If a dental dam is utilized in a pediatric crown prep, a smaller-sized dam, specifically designed for primary teeth, may be used.

5. Pulpotomy or Pulp Therapy Materials (Optional): In cases where the tooth has extensive decay or pulp involvement, a pulpotomy or pulp therapy may be performed before the crown preparation. Materials such as mineral trioxide aggregate (MTA) or formocresol may be used.

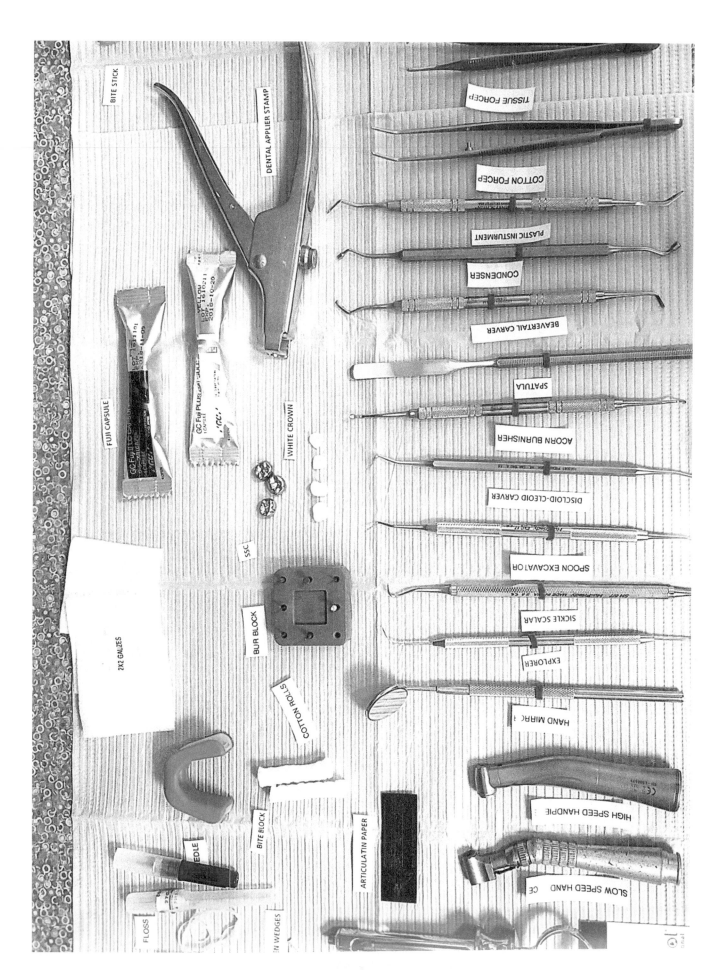

Extraction Tray: Before we dive into the details of a dental tray setup for an extraction procedure, it's important to note that the specific instruments used may vary slightly depending on the dentist's preference and the complexity of the extraction. However, I will provide you with a general overview of the instruments commonly found on a dental tray for this procedure.

1. Local Anesthetic Syringe: This syringe contains the anesthetic solution used to numb the area around the tooth that will be extracted. It typically consists of a barrel, plunger, and a needle. The dentist will use this instrument to administer the anesthetic to ensure a pain-free procedure.

2. Needle Holder: A needle holder is a handheld instrument designed to securely hold the needle during the administration of anesthetic. It facilitates proper control and precise maneuvering while minimizing the risk of needlestick injuries.

3. Dental Mirror: The dental mirror is a small, handheld instrument with a mirror attached at one end. It helps the dentist visualize hard-to-reach areas in the mouth, such as the posterior regions, to ensure optimal visibility during the extraction procedure.

4. Explorer: The explorer, often referred to as a dental probe, is a thin, long instrument with a sharp point at one end. It is primarily used to help identify cavities, detect tooth decay, and assess the stability of the tooth to be extracted.

5. Cotton Forceps: These forceps are used to handle cotton rolls or small pieces of cotton. During extraction, they are often used for moisture control by isolating the surgical area, ensuring a dry and clean environment.

6. Straight Elevator: A straight elevator is a handheld instrument with a flat, blunt end used to loosen the tooth from its socket before extraction. It is placed between the tooth and the surrounding bone structure and is used to apply controlled forces to elevate and luxate the tooth. Extraction Forceps:

7. Extraction forceps are used to grasp the tooth being extracted firmly. There are different types of forceps based on the specific tooth and their shape. For example, the most common forceps used for simple extractions is the Universal forceps, while anterior forceps are commonly used for incisors and canines.

8. Surgical Curette: A surgical curette is a handheld instrument with a sharp-edged, spoon- shaped tip that is used to remove any soft tissue debris or infected material

from the socket after extraction. It aids in cleaning and debriding the area to promote proper healing.

9. Suturing Instruments: Depending on the complexity of the extraction, the dental tray may also include suturing instruments like surgical needles and silk or resorbable sutures. These instruments are used to close the extraction site once the tooth has been removed. They aid in proper wound closure, reducing the risk of postoperative complications.

10. Scalpel: Used for making incisions when necessary.

11. Retractors: Used to hold the soft tissues away during the extraction procedure.

12. Rongeurs: Used for removing bone fragments, particularly for difficult or impacted extractions.

13. Surgical Aspirator: Used to remove blood, saliva, and debris from the oral12. cavity during the procedure.

14. Hemostatic Agents: Such as gelatin sponges or oxidized cellulose, used to aid in controlling bleeding.

It's essential to note that dental tray setups may also include additional instruments, such as dental drills or bone files, which may be necessary for more complex extractions. However, the instruments mentioned above form the foundational setup for a standard extraction procedure.

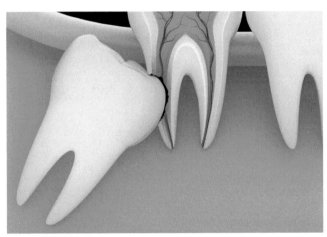

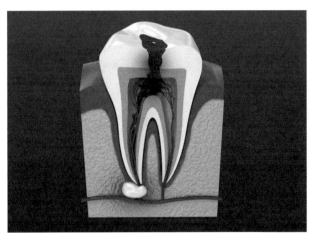

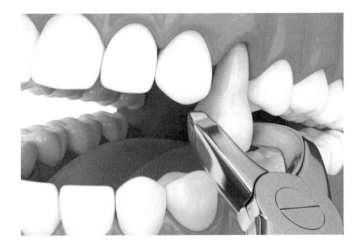

Student Clinics Extraction Setup Tray

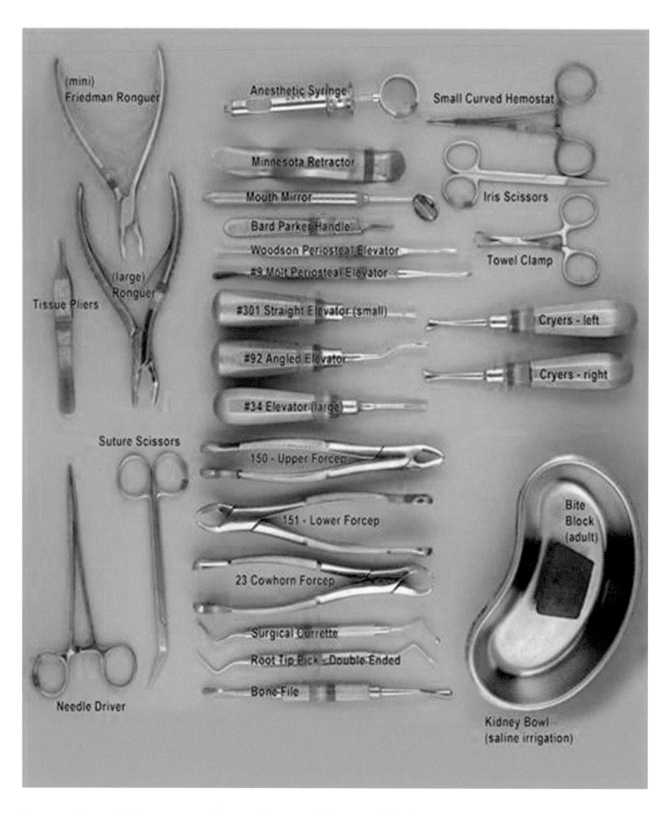

Remember, this is a general overview, and the specific instruments may vary depending on the dentist's preferences and the patient's individual needs.

Suture Removal

As a dental assistant, there are specific tasks and responsibilities
that you can perform, including suture removal.

Suture removal is a common procedure in dentistry, particularly after oral surgery or any other procedure that requires the use of stitches or sutures to close a wound. The purpose of removing sutures is to promote healing and prevent any potential complications.

Dental assistants can assist the dentist or oral surgeon during the suture removal process under their supervision. Depending on your state's dental practice act and the specific guidelines set by your dentist, you may also be able to perform suture removal on your own, as long as certain requirements are met.

To be qualified to perform suture removal as a dental assistant, you may need to:

1. Receive appropriate training: It is important to undergo proper training and education to understand the steps involved in suture removal, the different types of sutures, and how to handle and dispose of them correctly.

2. Gain experience: Hands-on experience under the supervision of a dentist or oral surgeon is crucial to becoming competent in suture removal. This experience will allow you to develop the necessary skills and confidence to perform the task effectively.

3. Know the regulations and protocols: Familiarize yourself with your state's dental practice act and the guidelines set by your dental office regarding suture removal. Ensure that you always follow appropriate infection control protocols and maintain a sterile environment during the procedure.

4. Communicate and collaborate with the dentist: Work closely with the dentist or oral surgeon during suture removal, follow their instructions, and seek clarification if needed. Open communication will ensure that the procedure is performed correctly and any complications are promptly addressed.

Remember, the scope of practice for dental assistants varies by state, and some states may have limitations on the tasks they can perform. It is essential to check with your state dental board or regulatory body to understand the specific requirements and regulations related to suture removal in your area.

Ultimately, with the right training, experience, and adherence to regulations, dental assistants can be a valuable asset in providing safe and efficient suture removal procedures in a dental office.

medical and dental history since their last visit and record any relevant information.

5. Providing Chairside support: During the cleaning procedure, you will assist the dentist or dental hygienist by passing instruments, suctioning excess water or saliva, and retracting the patient's cheek or tongue for better access to the teeth.

6. Dental charting: You may be responsible for charting the patient's oral health status, noting any dental decay, gum disease, or abnormalities observed during the cleaning process.

7. Polishing and applying fluoride: License Permitting Must be RDA You may assist in polishing the patient's teeth using a dental handpiece and pumice, and applying fluoride varnish or gel as directed by the dentist or dental hygienist.

8. Educating the patient: You will provide post-care instructions to the patient, including proper brushing and flossing techniques, the importance of regular dental visits, and suggestions for maintaining good oral health.

Throughout all these procedures, it's crucial to maintain strict infection control measures, provide exceptional patient care, and anticipate the dentist's needs to ensure smooth and effective treatment for the patient.

– Clear Communication: Learn effective communication techniques to anticipate the dentist's needs, provide relevant information, and assist in patient comfort.

Effective communication and the ability to anticipate the dentist's needs are essential skills for a dental assistant, especially for someone who is just starting in the field. Here are some tips to help you improve your communication skills and provide optimal assistance:

1. Active listening: Pay close attention to what the dentist is saying or asking for. Actively listen and focus on their instructions. This will help you anticipate their needs and respond quickly and accurately.

2. Clarifying questions: If you are unsure about a task or instruction, don't hesitate to ask for clarification. It's better to ask questions and ensure you have a clear understanding rather than making assumptions that may lead to mistakes.

3. Anticipating tools and materials: Familiarize yourself with the different instruments and materials used in various procedures. Anticipate which tools and materials the dentist may require next, and have them prepared and ready for use.

4. Non-verbal cues: Pay attention to the dentist's body language, facial expressions, and gestures. These cues can provide valuable information about their needs, preferences, and level of comfort. Anticipate their needs by promptly responding to these cues. Medical and dental history since their last visit and record any relevant information.

5. Providing Chairside support: During the cleaning procedure, you will assist the dentist or dental hygienist by passing instruments, suctioning excess water or saliva, and retracting the patient's cheek or tongue for better access to the teeth.

6. Dental charting: You may be responsible for charting the patient's oral health status, noting any dental decay, gum disease, or abnormalities observed during the cleaning process.

7. Polishing and applying fluoride: License Permitting Must be RDA You may assist in polishing the patient's teeth using a dental handpiece and pumice, and applying fluoride varnish or gel as directed by the dentist or dental hygienist.

8. Educating the patient: You will provide post-care instructions to the patient, including proper brushing and flossing techniques, the importance of regular dental visits, and suggestions for maintaining good oral health.

Throughout all these procedures, it's crucial to maintain strict infection control measures, provide exceptional patient care, and anticipate the dentist's needs to ensure smooth and effective treatment for the patient.

– Clear Communication: Learn effective communication techniques to anticipate the dentist's needs, provide relevant information, and assist in patient comfort.

Effective communication and the ability to anticipate the dentist's needs are essential skills for a dental assistant, especially for someone who is just starting in the field.

Here are some tips to help you improve your communication skills and provide optimal assistance:

1. Active listening: Pay close attention to what the dentist is saying or asking for. Actively listen and focus on their instructions. This will help you anticipate their needs and respond quickly and accurately.

2. Clarifying questions: If you are unsure about a task or instruction, don't hesitate to ask for clarification. It's better to ask questions and ensure you have a clear understanding rather than making assumptions that may lead to mistakes.

3. Anticipating tools and materials: Familiarize yourself with the different instruments and materials used in various procedures. Anticipate which tools and materials the dentist may require next, and have them prepared and ready for use.

4. Non-verbal cues: Pay attention to the dentist's body language, facial expressions, and gestures. These cues can provide valuable information about their needs, preferences, and level of comfort. Anticipate their needs by promptly responding to these cues.

Suture Tray Set- Up

- **Mouth Mirror**
- **2X2 Gauze**
- **Cotton Rolls**
- **Hemostat**
- **Suture Scissors**
- **Cotton Forcep**
- **Suture and Needle**

Suture Removal Tray Set-Up

- **Explorer/ Perioprobe**
- **Mouth Mirror**
- **Cotton Forcep**
- **Suture Scissors**
- **Cotton Rolls**
- **2X2 Gauzes**

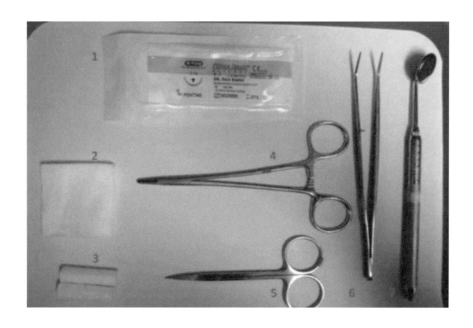

LESSON 10

Directing Dentists during Procedures:

Chairside Assistance:

As a dental assistant, your role is crucial in providing chairside assistance to the dentist during various dental procedures. Your responsibilities will vary depending on the specific procedure being performed, but here is a detailed breakdown of the essential tasks you may be involved in during fillings, extractions, and cleaning procedures:

Fillings:

1. **Preparing the treatment area** P: Before the filling procedure, you will ensure that the treatment room is ready. This includes ensuring that all necessary instruments and materials are set up, the dental chair is adjusted properly, and the patient is comfortably seated.

2. Assisting with patient communication: You will greet the patient, explain the procedure, and answer any questions or concerns they may have. It's important to maintain a calm and reassuring demeanor to help alleviate any anxiety.

3. Taking and recording patient history: You will review the patient's medical and dental history, noting any relevant information such as allergies or medical conditions that may affect the treatment.

4. Preparing the patient: You will drape the patient with a protective covering and provide them with protective eyewear. This ensures their safety and minimizes the spread of infection.

5. Providing Chairside support: During the filling procedure, you will assist the dentist by passing instruments, suctioning excess water or saliva from the patient's mouth, and retracting the patient's cheek or tongue to ensure clear visibility for the dentist.

6. Mixing dental materials: Depending on the type of filling, you may be responsible for mixing dental materials such as dental composites, amalgam, or Glass Ionomer Cement (GIC).

7. Obtaining dental radiographs: You may assist in taking dental radiographs (X-rays) to help the dentist diagnose and assess the extent of the tooth decay or damage before the filling procedure.

8. Infection control: Throughout the procedure, you will adhere to strict infection control protocols. This involves wearing personal protective equipment (PPE) such as gloves, masks, and eyewear, as well as proper handling and disposal of contaminated materials.

Extractions:

1. Preparing the treatment area: Just like with fillings, you will set up the treatment room and ensure all necessary instruments and materials are ready.

2. Assisting with patient communication: Similar to fillings, you will communicate and educate the patient about the extraction procedure, answer their questions, and ensure they are comfortable and at ease.

3. Preparing the patient: You will drape the patient with a protective covering, provide them with protective eyewear, and make sure they are in a comfortable position.

4. Providing Chairside support: During extractions, you will assist the dentist by passing instruments, suctioning excess saliva or blood from the oral cavity, and retracting the patient's cheek or tongue to improve visibility.

5. Taking dental radiographs: license Permitting: You may assist in taking dental radiographs to aid the dentist in assessing the tooth or teeth to be extracted.

6. Maintaining proper suction: It is important to keep the treatment area clean and visible by operating high-volume suction during the extraction procedure to remove excess saliva, blood, and debris from the oral cavity.

7. Assisting with hemostasis: After the tooth extraction, you may assist the dentist in controlling bleeding by placing gauze or instructing the patient on how to bite down on a gauze pad for a certain duration.

8. Post-operative instructions: You may be responsible for providing the patient with post-operative care instructions, including proper oral hygiene practices, diet restrictions, and information on managing any discomfort or swelling.

Cleanings:

1. Preparing the treatment area: Similar to other procedures, you will ensure the treatment room is set up appropriately, including having the necessary instruments and materials ready.

2. Assisting with patient communication: As with other procedures, you will communicate with the patient, explain the cleaning process, address any concerns they may have, and ensure they feel comfortable.

3. Preparing the patient: You will help the patient get settled in the dental chair, provide them with protective eyewear, and ensure they are relaxed before the cleaning begins.

4. Taking and recording patient history: You will inquire about any changes in the patient's medical and dental history since their last visit and record any relevant information.

5. Providing Chairside support: During the cleaning procedure, you will assist the dentist or dental hygienist by passing instruments, suctioning excess water or saliva, and retracting the patient's cheek or tongue for better access to the teeth.

6. Dental charting: You may be responsible for charting the patient's oral health status, noting any dental decay, gum disease, or abnormalities observed during the cleaning process.

7. Polishing and applying fluoride: License Permitting Must be RDA You may assist in polishing the patient's teeth using a dental handpiece and pumice, and applying fluoride varnish or gel as directed by the dentist or dental hygienist.

8. Educating the patient: You will provide post-care instructions to the patient, including proper brushing and flossing techniques, the importance of regular dental visits, and suggestions for maintaining good oral health.

Throughout all these procedures, it's crucial to maintain strict infection control measures, provide exceptional patient care, and anticipate the dentist's needs to ensure smooth and effective treatment for the patient.

- Clear Communication: Learn effective communication techniques to anticipate the dentist's needs, provide relevant information, and assist in patient comfort.

Effective communication and the ability to anticipate the dentist's needs are essential skills for a dental assistant, especially for someone who is just starting in the field. Here are some tips to help you improve your communication skills and provide optimal assistance:

1. Active listening: Pay close attention to what the dentist is saying or asking for. Actively listen and focus on their instructions. This will help you anticipate their needs and respond quickly and accurately.

2. Clarifying questions: If you are unsure about a task or instruction, don't hesitate to ask for clarification. It's better to ask questions and ensure you have a clear understanding rather than making assumptions that may lead to mistakes.

3. Anticipating tools and materials: Familiarize yourself with the different instruments and materials used in various procedures. Anticipate which tools and materials the dentist may require next, and have them prepared and ready for use.

4. Non-verbal cues: Pay attention to the dentist's body language, facial expressions, and gestures. These cues can provide valuable information about their needs, preferences, and level of comfort. Anticipate their needs by promptly responding to these cues.

5. Efficient instrument passing: Learn the proper techniques for passing instruments to the dentist. Hand instruments in a manner that allows the dentist to grasp them easily and without disruption to the procedure. Be mindful of the dentist's hand preferences, whether they are left-handed or right-handed.

6. Clear and concise communication: When providing information to the dentist, use clear and concise language. Avoid using ambiguous terms or jargon that may cause confusion. Present information in a logical and organized manner.

7. Proactive chairside assistance: Anticipate the steps of the procedure and be proactive in providing assistance. For example, have suction ready to remove excess saliva or water, or have a mirror and retractor available to maintain clear visibility for the dentist.

8. Patient comfort: Pay attention to the patient's comfort throughout the procedure. Communicate with the patient to ensure they are feeling comfortable and inform the dentist if the patient needs any adjustments or breaks.

9. Empathy and emotional support: Dental procedures can sometimes be stressful for patients. Show empathy, offer words of encouragement, and provide emotional support to help alleviate their anxiety. Build a rapport with patients to make them feel more at ease during their dental visits.

10. Teamwork and collaboration: Communication with other dental staff members, such as dental hygienists or receptionists, is crucial for ensuring a smooth workflow. Collaborate effectively, provide updates as necessary, and be willing to assist others when needed. Remember, effective communication skills improve with practice and experience. Emphasize professionalism, active listening, and clear communication to anticipate the dentist's needs, provide relevant information, and ensure optimal patient comfort.

LESSON 11

Behavior Management

Understanding the unique needs of both children and adults in a dental setting is crucial for providing effective care. While it is true that many anxiety issues may stem from childhood, it's important to remember that adults can also suffer from anxiety. So, let's dive into how we can address anxiety in patients of all ages while adding a touch of humor along the way!

When it comes to managing anxiety in both children and adults, humor can be a powerful tool. Incorporating jokes, funny stories, or even silly props can help create a more relaxed and lighthearted atmosphere. Laughter not only helps to reduce anxiety, but it also builds rapport and trust between the dental team and the patient.

Now, let's talk about the techniques that can be used to manage anxiety in both kids and adults. For children, using techniques like tell-show-do can be really effective. This involves explaining the procedure in a child-friendly way, showing them the tools before using them, and then carrying out the procedure. But let's not forget, even adults can benefit from a little "tell-show-do" action too! It helps to demystify the procedure and reduce anxiety.

Positive reinforcement and distractions are also important for managing anxiety in both children and adults. Offering praise, small rewards, or even a sticker chart for adults (who doesn't love stickers, right?) can motivate and encourage cooperation. And for those who prefer a little distraction, why not have a TV show or some soothing music playing in the background? It can help divert their attention and ease their anxiety.

Addressing dental fear and phobias is crucial, and using humor can be a great way to do it. Incorporating funny names for dental tools or making light-hearted jokes can help to ease tension and make the experience more enjoyable. Of course, it's important to gauge each patient's response and ensure that humor is used in a way that is comfortable and appropriate for them.

When it comes to treating patients with special needs, it is essential to approach each individual with sensitivity and adaptability. Using humor to create a relaxed and comfortable environment can be especially beneficial for these patients. Tailoring communication strategies and treatment plans to meet their specific needs, while still injecting some humor, can make a world of difference.

Now, let's talk about our adult patients. Dental anxiety is no joke, and it's important to address their fears and concerns in a compassionate and light-hearted manner. Explaining procedures step-by-step, using visual aids, and creating a calm and soothing environment can help ease their anxiety.

And don't forget to sprinkle in some humor along the way to lighten the mood! Active listening and empathy are also key when treating anxious adult patients. Taking the time to listen to their concerns and fears, offering reassurance, and acknowledging their anxieties can go a long way in making them feel more at ease. And hey, if a well-timed joke or funny story can bring a smile to their face, that's even better!

Finally, if necessary, collaborating with the dentist to explore sedation or anesthesia options can be a game-changer for highly anxious adult patients. Providing them with options that will help minimize their discomfort and fear can make all the difference in their dental experience.

Remember, treating patients of all ages requires understanding, compassion, and a touch of humor. By implementing these strategies and creating a relaxed and fun environment, dental assistants can help patients overcome their anxiety and have a positive dental experience. So, let's bring on the laughs and create a truly patient-centered and enjoyable dental journey for everyone!

Special needs and disorders you might encounter in dentistry and tips on how to manage patients with these disorders:

1. Autism Spectrum Disorder (ASD): Patients with ASD may have difficulty with sensory sensitivities, communication, and social interactions. It is important to create a calm and structured environment for these patients. Using visual aids or social stories can help prepare them for dental visits. Be patient and provide clear, concise instructions. Consider using alternative behavior management techniques such as tell-show-do or desensitization techniques.

2. Down Syndrome: Individuals with Down Syndrome may have delayed tooth eruption, missing teeth, or abnormal tooth structure. They may also have cognitive impairments and reduced muscle tone. Adapt your communication style by using simple language and visual aids. Offer frequent breaks if needed and allow extra time for appointments. Regular dental check-ups are crucial to monitor any oral health issues that may arise.

3. Cerebral Palsy Patients with cerebral palsy may control, and mobility. Adjust the dental chair to accommodate their positioning needs and ensure their safety during treatment. Use a gentle touch and provide support as needed. Communication may be challenging, so be patient and use alternative communication methods if necessary.

4. Intellectual Disabilities: Patients with intellectual disabilities may have varying cognitive impairments and communication difficulties. Establish trust and rapport through positive reinforcement and praise. Use alternative communication methods such as pictures or gestures. Break procedures down into simpler steps and provide frequent breaks. Remember to involve caregivers or family members in treatment planning.

5. Attention Deficit Hyperactivity Disorder (ADHD): Patients with ADHD may have difficulty with attention, impulsivity, and hyperactivity. Create a structured and predictable dental environment to minimize distractions. eep instructions clear and concise. Consider shorter appointment times and breaks if needed. Positive reinforcement and rewards can help keep the patient engaged.

6. Sensory Processing Disorder (SPD): Patients with SPD may have heightened or diminished responses to sensory stimuli, making some dental procedures challenging. Create a comfortable environment by minimizing bright lights, loud noises, and strong smells. Use adaptive equipment such as weighted blankets or headphones if needed. Gradually introduce unfamiliar sensations to desensitize the patient.

It is important to note that each patient is unique, and their needs may vary. Collaborate with their caregivers, healthcare professionals, and specialists to create an individualized treatment plan that addresses their specific needs and ensures their comfort and safety during dental visits.

LESSON 12

Dental Assistant Responsibilities - Charting

Introduction:

In this chapter, we will explore the crucial responsibility of dental assistants when it comes to charting. Charting is a vital aspect of dental care that involves accurately recording and documenting a patient's oral health information. It helps the dental team keep track of a patient's dental history, treatment plans, and progress. Let's dive into the detailed and in - depth process of charting, including what to chart, how to chart, and common abbreviations used.

1. Importance of Charting:

Charting plays a crucial role in maintaining comprehensive dental records. It provides a visual representation of a patient's oral health status, allowing dentists, hygienists, and other dental professionals to assess, plan, and deliver appropriate dental care. Accurate charting ensures continuity of care, facilitates communication among dental team members, and assists in making informed treatment decisions.

2. What to Chart:

To create a comprehensive oral health record, dental assistants should chart the following:

   a. Existing and new restorations: Documenting the location, type (e.g., amalgam, composite), and condition of restorations.
   b. Missing teeth: Indicate the teeth that are absent and note the reason (e.g., extraction, congenital absence).
   c. Periodontal measurements: Recording pocket depths, bleeding points, and other periodontal findings.
   d. Oral pathology: Document any notable abnormalities, lesions, or growths observed during examinations.
   e. Treatment plans: Including planned or completed procedures, such as fillings, extractions, or orthodontic treatments.
   f. Radiographic findings: Noting any abnormalities or observed pathologies found in dental X-rays.

g. Patient notes: Documenting relevant information like patient complaints, concerns, or specific instructions provided.

3. Charting Techniques:

Dental assistants use various charting techniques to accurately and efficiently record information. The preferred methods include:

a. Anatomical Charting: Using tooth diagrams to mark restorations, missing teeth, and any other pertinent observations with various abbreviations used in dental charting. Some common abbreviations include:

1. FMX - Full Mouth X-rays: Refers to a complete set of dental X-rays, typically taken at the initial visit or during a comprehensive examination.
2. P - Permanent: Indicates a permanent tooth.
3. E - Eruption: Indicates the stage of tooth eruption.
4. M - Missing: Indicates a missing tooth.
5. O - Extracted: Indicates a tooth that has been extracted or removed.
6. C - Caries: Indicates tooth decay or cavities.
7. F - Filling: Indicates a tooth that has been restored with a filling material.
8. RCT - Root Canal Treatment: Indicates a tooth that has received root canal therapy.
9. PD - Periodontal Disease: Indicates a tooth or area affected by gum disease.
10. B/L - Buccal/Lingual: Indicates the surface of the tooth facing the cheek (buccal) or tongue (lingual).
11. ADA - American Dental Association: The professional association of dentists in the United States.
12. DDS - Doctor of Dental Surgery: The degree awarded to dentists who have completed dental school.
13. DMD - Doctor of Dental Medicine: An alternative degree to DDS, both reflecting the same education and qualifications.
14. DENT - Dentistry: The field of medicine that focuses on oral health and the treatment of teeth and gums.
15. OHI - Oral Health Instructions: Guidance provided by dental professionals on maintaining good oral hygiene.
16. PPE - Personal Protective Equipment: Equipment worn to protect dental professionals and patients from potential hazards.
17. OTC - Over-the-counter: Refers to dental products available for purchase without a prescription, such as toothpaste or mouthwash.

18. TMJ - Temporomandibular Joint: The joint connecting the jawbone to the skull. TMJ disorders can cause pain and dysfunction.
19. BPE - Basic Periodontal Examination: A screening tool used to assess periodontal health and diagnose gum diseases.
20. OCCLUSAL - Referring to the chewing surface of teeth, particularly used when describing dental procedures or restorations.
21. MO - Mesio-Occlusal: This refers to the surface between the mesial and occlusal surfaces of a tooth.
22. DO - Disto-Occlusal: This refers to the surface between the distal and occlusal surfaces of a tooth.
23. MOD - Mesio-Occlusal-Distal: This refers to the combination of all three surfaces: mesial, occlusal, and distal.
24. DL: Distal Lingual (refers to the surface of a tooth between the distal and lingual aspects)
25. FDI: Fédération Dentaire Internationale (international notation system for tooth numbering)
26. PD: Pocket Depth (measurement in millimeters from the gingival margin to the base of the pocket)
27. BOP: Bleeding On Probing (indicator of potential periodontal disease)

Charting is an essential responsibility of dental assistants as it helps create a comprehensive record of a patient's oral health. By accurately documenting information through proper charting techniques and utilizing common abbreviations, dental assistants contribute to effective communication, continuity of care, and informed treatment decisions. Mastering charting skills will not only enhance your professional capabilities but also ensure the provision of high-quality dental care to your patients.

LESSON 13

Chairside Dental Assistant Study Guide Practice test and study guide

1. What is the primary purpose of sterilization in the dental field?
   a) To minimize cross-contamination
   b) To reduce patient discomfort
   c) To improve dental aesthetics
   d) To increase treatment efficiency

2. How does effective sterilization practices contribute to dental professionalism?
   a) By reducing treatment costs
   b) By ensuring patient comfort
   c) By establishing trust and professionalism
   d) By enhancing treatment outcomes

3. Which of the following is an important aspect of managing sterilized dental products?
   a) Maintaining sterilization logs
   b) Increasing production speed
   c) Using expired sterilized items
   d) Ignoring recommended storage guidelines

4. What are some commonly used chemicals for dental sterilization?
   a) Autoclave and hand sanitizers
   b) Hand sanitizers and surface disinfectants
   c) Autoclave and surface disinfectants
   d) Chemical sterilants and hand sanitizers

5. Which organization has specific requirements for sterilization in dental offices?
   a) ADA (American Dental Association)
   b) CDC (Centers for Disease Control and Prevention)
   c) OSHA (Occupational Safety and Health Administration)
   d) EPA (Environmental Protection Agency)

6. What should be done with contaminated instruments after use?
   a) Dispose of them in regular trash bins
   b) Store them in a designated area for reuse
   c) Place them back in cassettes for sterilization
   d) Clean them with soap and water for immediate reuse

7. What is the recommended cleaning protocol for operatory breakdown?
   a) Start cleaning from the cleanest area
   b) Clean protective eyewear first
   c) Disinfect heavy-duty gloves before cleaning
   d) Clean the patient chair last

8. What should be done to ensure effective disinfection during operatory cleaning?
   a) Apply disinfectant spray and immediately wipe it off
   b) Use cleaning products not recommended by the office
   c) Keep treated areas dry for a longer time
   d) Follow the required contact time for disinfection

9. How should heavy-duty gloves be cleaned during operatory breakdown?
   a) Use a suitable cleaning product to clean the gloves
   b) Dispose of the gloves in the designated sharps container
   c) Rinse the gloves with warm water and air dry
   d) Skip cleaning the gloves to save time

10. What is the recommended practice for flushing air and water lines in the operatory?
   a) Flush for 2 minutes between each patient
   b) Flush for 20 seconds at the start of each day
   c) Flush for 30 seconds after each procedure
   d) Flush for 1 minute before and after each patient

Beginning of the Day:

11. Check and replenish dental supplies (e.g., gloves, masks, sterilization pouches): Ensure availability for daily procedures.
   a) Gloves and masks
   b) Sterilization pouches
   c) Both a) and b)
   d) None of the above

12. Clean and disinfect treatment chairs and surfaces: Maintain infection control and patient safety.
   a) Once a week
   b) Every other day
   c) Every day
   d) Only when visibly dirty

13. Prepare dental unit water bottle and flush lines: Ensure proper water supply for procedures.
    a) Flush lines with cleane
    b) Fill water bottles with distilled water
    c) Both a) and b)
    d) None of the above

End of the Day:

14. Clean and disinfect handpieces: Prevent cross-contamination and maintain hygiene.
    a) Once a month
    b) Once a week
    c) Every day
    d) Only when requested by a patient

15. Empty and clean amalgam separator: Prevent waste buildup and maintain suction efficiency.
    a) Once a year
    b) Every 6 months
    c) Every month
    d) Every day

16. Turn off and unplug equipment: Reduce energy consumption and minimize hazards.
    a) Only unplug equipment
    b) Only turn off equipment
    c) Both unplug and turn off equipment
    d) None of the above

Weekly Maintenance:

17. Check and clean handpieces: Ensure proper functionality and prevent cross-contamination.
    a) Once a month
    b) Once a week
    c) Every day
    d) Only when requested by a patient

18. Inspect and clean suction system filters: Maintain proper suction and prevent clogs.
    a) Once a month
    b) Once a week

c) Every day

d) Only when visibly dirty

19. Check and clean autoclave: Ensure effective sterilization and prevent infections.
    a) Once a month
    b) Once a week
    c) Every day
    d) Only when requested by a patient

20. Inspect waterlines and flush with appropriate cleaning solution: Maintain water quality and prevent biofilm buildup.
    a) Once a month
    b) Once a week
    c) Every day
    d) Only when visibly dirty

Tooth Structure:

21. What is the outermost layer of the tooth's crown?
    a) Root
    b) Dentin
    c) Enamel
    d) Pulp

22. Which part of the tooth provides support and strength?
    a) Crown
    b) Pulp
    c) Dentin
    d) Enamel

23. Where is the dental pulp located?
    a) In the center of the tooth
    b) On the root surface of the tooth
    c) Beneath the enamel
    d) Surrounding the tooth in the jawbone

24. What is the specialized bone that surrounds and supports the teeth?
    a) Pulp
    b) Cementum

c) Periodontal ligament

d) Alveolar bone

Tooth Numbering Systems:

25. Which tooth numbering system assigns a number to each tooth, starting from the upper right third molar?
    a) Universal Numbering System
    b) Palmer Notation Method
    c) Both a) and b)
    d) None of the above

26. How is the upper right second molar represented in the Palmer Notation Method?
    a) UR1
    b) UR2
    c) UR6
    d) UR7

27. When did four-handed dentistry begin to be practiced?
    a) 1960
    b) 1970
    c) 20th century
    d) 1990

28. What is one benefit of four-handed dentistry?
    a) Increased waiting times
    b) Reduced efficiency in dental procedures
    c) Improved speed and efficiency
    d) Increased physical stress on the dentist

29. How does four-handed dentistry help enhance patient comfort and safety?
    a) By causing errors and discomfort for the patient
    b) By minimizing strain on individual muscles
    c) By reducing access to the treatment area
    d) By reducing the need for dental assistants

30. What is hand-over-hand instrument technique also known as?
    a) Dental assisting programs
    b) Streamlined dental treatment

c) Four-handed dentistry

d) Coordinated movements

31. What is the primary purpose of sterilization in the dental field?
    a) To minimize cross-contamination
    b) To reduce patient discomfort
    c) To improve dental aesthetics
    d) To increase treatment efficiency

32. How does effective sterilization practices contribute to dental professionalism?
    a) By reducing treatment costs
    b) By ensuring patient comfort
    c) By establishing trust and professionalism
    d) By enhancing treatment outcomes

33. Which of the following is an important aspect of managing sterilized dental products?
    a) Maintaining sterilization logs
    b) Increasing production speed
    c) Using expired sterilized items

34. Ignoring recommended storage guidelines

35. What are some commonly used chemicals for dental sterilization?
    a) Autoclave and hand sanitizers
    b) Hand sanitizers and surface disinfectants
    c) Autoclave and surface disinfectants
    d) Chemical sterilants and hand sanitizers

36. Which organization has specific requirements for sterilization in dental offices?
    a) ADA (American Dental Association)
    b) CDC (Centers for Disease Control and Prevention)
    c) OSHA (Occupational Safety and Health Administration)
    d) EPA (Environmental Protection Agency)

37. What should be done with contaminated instruments after use?
    a) Dispose of them in regular trash bins
    b) Store them in a designated area for reuse
    c) Place them back in cassettes for sterilization
    d) Clean them with soap and water for immediate reuse

38. What is the recommended cleaning protocol for operatory breakdown?
    a) Start cleaning from the cleanest area
    b) Clean protective eyewear first
    c) Disinfect heavy-duty gloves before cleaning
    d) Clean the patient chair last

39. What should be done to ensure effective disinfection during operatory cleaning?
    a) Apply disinfectant spray and immediately wipe it off
    b) Use cleaning products not recommended by the office
    c) Keep treated areas dry for a longer time
    d) Follow the required contact time for disinfection

40. How should heavy-duty gloves be cleaned during operatory breakdown?
    a) Use a suitable cleaning product to clean the gloves
    b) Dispose of the gloves in the designated sharps container
    c) Rinse the gloves with warm water and air dry
    d) Skip cleaning the gloves to save time

41. What is the recommended practice for flushing air and water lines in the operatory?
    a) Flush for 2 minutes between each patient
    b) Flush for 20 seconds at the start of each day
    c) Flush for 30 seconds after each procedure
    d) Flush for 1 minute before and after each patient

Answers

1. What is the primary purpose of sterilization in the dental field?
   Answer: a) To minimize cross-contamination

2. How does effective sterilization practices contribute to dental professionalism?
   Answer: c) By establishing trust and professionalism

3. Which of the following is an important aspect of managing sterilized dental products?
   Answer: a) Maintaining sterilization logs

4. What are some commonly used chemicals for dental sterilization?
   Answer: d) Chemical sterilants and hand sanitizers

5. Which organization has specific requirements for sterilization in dental offices?
   Answer: c) OSHA (Occupational Safety and Health Administration)

6. What should be done with contaminated instruments after use?
   Answer: c) Place them back in cassettes for sterilization

7. What is the recommended cleaning protocol for operatory breakdown?
   Answer: a) Start cleaning from the cleanest area

8. What should be done to ensure effective disinfection during operatory cleaning?
   Answer: d) Follow the required contact time for disinfection

9. How should heavy-duty gloves be cleaned during operatory breakdown?
   Answer: a) Use a suitable cleaning product to clean the gloves

10. What is the recommended practice for flushing air and water lines in the operatory?
    Answer: b) Flush for 20 seconds at the start of each day

Beginning of the Day:

11. Check and replenish dental supplies (e.g., gloves, masks, sterilization pouches): Ensure availability for daily procedures.
    Answer: c) Both a) and b) - Gloves and masks, and sterilization pouches.

12. Clean and disinfect treatment chairs and surfaces: Maintain infection control and patient safety.
    Answer: c) Every day

13. Prepare dental unit water bottle and flush lines: Ensure proper water supply for procedures.
    Answer: a) Flush lines with cleaner

End of the Day:

14. Clean and disinfect handpieces: Prevent cross-contamination and ensure proper functioning.
    Answer: c) Every day

15. Empty and clean amalgam separator: Prevent amalgam waste buildup and maintain suction system efficacy.
    Answer: c) Every month

16. Turn off and unplug equipment: Reduce energy consumption and prevent hazards.
    Answer: c) Both unplug and turn off equipment

Weekly Maintenance

17. Check and clean handpieces: Ensure proper functionality and prevent cross-contamination.
    Answer: b) Once a week

18. Inspect and clean suction system filters: Maintain proper suction and prevent clogs.
    Answer: b) Once a week

19. Check and clean autoclave: Ensure effective sterilization and prevent infections.
    Answer: a) Once a month

20. Inspect waterlines and flush with appropriate cleaning solution: Maintain water quality and prevent biofilm buildup.
    Answer: b) Once a week

Tooth Structure:

21. What is the outermost layer of the tooth's crown?
    Answer: c) Enamel

22. Which part of the tooth provides support and strength?
    Answer: c) Dentin

23. Where is the dental pulp located?
    Answer: a) In the center of the tooth

24. What is the specialized bone that surrounds and supports the teeth?
    Answer: d) Alveolar bone

Tooth Numbering Systems:

25. Which tooth numbering system assigns a number to each tooth, starting from the upper right third molar?
    Answer: a) Universal Numbering System

26. How is the upper right second molar represented in the Palmer Notation Method?
    Answer: d) UR7

Answers

27. When did four-handed dentistry begin to be practiced?
    Answer: c) 20th century

28. What is one benefit of four-handed dentistry?
    Answer: c) Improved speed and efficiency

29. How does four-handed dentistry help enhance patient comfort and safety?
    Answer: b) By minimizing strain on individual muscles and d) By reducing the likelihood of errors and discomfort for the patient

30. What is hand-over-hand instrument technique also known as?
    Answer: c) Four-handed dentistry

31. What is the primary purpose of sterilization in the dental field?
    Answer: a) To minimize cross-contamination

32. How does effective sterilization practices contribute to dental professionalism?
    Answer: c) By establishing trust and professionalism

33. Which of the following is an important aspect of managing sterilized dental products?
    Answer: a) Maintaining sterilization logs

34. What are some commonly used chemicals for dental sterilization?
    Answer: d) Chemical sterilants and hand sanitizers

35. Which organization has specific requirements for sterilization in dental offices?
    Answer: c) OSHA (Occupational Safety and Health Administration)

36. What should be done with contaminated instruments after use?
    Answer: c) Place them back in cassettes for sterilization

37. What is the recommended cleaning protocol for operatory breakdown?
    Answer: a) Start cleaning from the cleanest area

38. What should be done to ensure effective disinfection during operatory cleaning?
    Answer: d) Follow the required contact time for disinfection

39. How should heavy-duty gloves be cleaned during operatory breakdown?
    Answer: a) Use a suitable cleaning product to clean the gloves

40. What is the recommended practice for flushing air and water lines in the operatory?
    Answer: b) Flush for 20 seconds at the start of each day

Dental Professional Resources: Prominent Outlets and Organization

1. California Dental Board: Regulates dental professionals in California. You can find their contact information on their official website.**www.dbc.ca.gov**

2. American Dental Association (ADA): A professional association for dentists in the United States. They provide resources, guidelines, and information on dental practices. You can visit their website for contact information. **www.ada.org**

3. Occupational Safety and Health Administration (OSHA): A federal agency that sets and enforces workplace safety standards. They provide guidelines and regulations relevant to dental offices. You can find OSHA's contact information on their official website. **Www.osha.com**

4. Centers for Disease Control and Prevention (CDC): Provides information and guidelines on infection control and other aspects of dental health. Their website is a valuable resource for research and best practices. Certainly! Here's a list of reputable outlets and organizations related to dentistry: **www.cdc.gov**

5. Academy of General Dentistry (AGD): An organization that promotes the professional development and continuing education of general dentists.**www.agd.org**

6. International Association for Dental Research (IADR): An organization dedicated to promoting research in oral health and dentistry worldwide.

7. American Academy of Pediatric Dentistry (AAPD): An organization focused on promoting oral health for children and advancing the specialty of pediatric dentistry.

8. American Association of Endodontists (AAE): A professional association representing endodontists and providing resources on root canal treatment and related procedures.

9. American Association of Orthodontists (AAO): An organization dedicated to advancing the field of orthodontics and promoting quality orthodontic care.

10. American Association of Oral and Maxillofacial Surgeons (AAOMS): An organization representing oral and maxillofacial surgeons and providing information on surgical procedures involving the mouth, jaws, and face.

11. American Dental Hygienists' Association (ADHA): An organization focused on advancing the dental hygiene profession and promoting oral health.

12. Dental Tribune: An online news source covering the latest developments, research, and trends in dentistry.

13. Journal of the American Dental Association (JADA): A peer-reviewed publication that publishes research articles, clinical studies, and other relevant information in dentistry.

As you embark on your professional journey, always remember the impact you can have on people's lives. Each patient is unique, and you have the power to create smiles and improve oral health. Approach every interaction with empathy, kindness, and expertise.

May your hands be steady, your mind sharp, and your heart compassionate. May you continue to seek knowledge, embrace innovation, and strive for excellence in every aspect of your practice. Remember that the pursuit of excellence never ends – it is a lifelong commitment.

Congratulations on reaching the end of this manual. You are now equipped with the tools and knowledge to make a difference in the world of dentistry. Embrace the challenges, embrace the opportunities, and always aim for excellence.

Wishing you all a successful and fulfilling journey ahead.

With warm regards,

:Corina-Dean; .McCabe-Jones:
corinajones.cj@gmail.com

Printed in the United States
by Baker & Taylor Publisher Services